The Therapy of Sound

Clederson Paduani

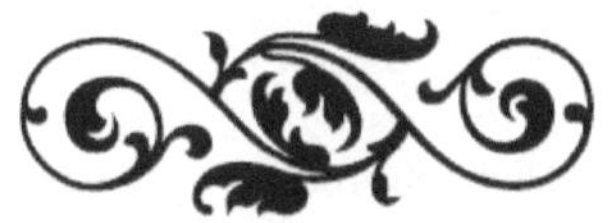

Florianópolis

2019

Dados Internacionais de Catalogação na Publicação (CIP)
Agência Brasileira do ISBN - Bibliotecária Priscila Pena Machado CRB-7/6971

```
P125   Paduani, Clederson.
           The therapy of sound / Clederson Paduani. —
       Florianópolis : Edição do autor, 2019.
           179 p. ; 21 cm.

           ISBN 978-65-900959-2-3

           1. Musicoterapia. 2. Energia vital - Uso terapêutico.
       3. Vibração. I. Título.


                                               CDD 615.851
```


Editorial Prefix: 900959
ISBN: 978-65-900959-2-3
Title: The Therapy of Sound

Cover: Ana Laura Daldegan Paduani.
Florianópolis - SC – Brazil.

I dedicate this book to my wife Ana Maria and my children, Victor and Ana Laura. Besides all their love, they also taught me everything I learned about what is most important in life.

PREFACE

Music is an art form in which a person can express his/her emotions in subtle ways, impregnated with feelings, using sound to conduct a strong affective appeal. It allows one to connect with the surroundings, which somehow participate in all the complexity and subtlety of the forms of expressions in real time. The sound vibrations conduce a movement coordinated by the performer directly to the ambiance, which perceives the sonic layout of a musical work orchestrated with all the harmony of whims elaborated by the author, driven by his sensitivity, and enriched by the contributions from all participating in the creative moment of a musical event.

The musical expression, whether performed simply by voice, individually, or orchestrated with a variety of instruments by a group, introduces an extraordinary *richness* of nuances made possible by the mixing of tonalities, timbres, and harmony of the notes produced. These, coming from different sources, such as voices or instruments, are tempered by the singular expression of each performer, who contributes with his/her particular sensitivity in the creation of the vibrant ambiance. Hence, a musical atmosphere comes up impregnated with feelings, touching the hearts of the listeners with the power to sensitize everyone in a peculiar and very personal way.

Music is thus an art form and a way of expression of the human unconscious, where one seeks to imbue sounds and words with feelings. The connotation of enchantment we can experience when hearing good music allows us to enjoy pleasant moments and a milder mood, as we thus become more susceptible to happiness. The good vibes we feel end up also spreading around, inducing a beneficial effect on everything in the surroundings. Music manifests itself as a subtle mechanism that allows us to achieve sublimation by providing moments of exacerbated sensitivity, good disposition, well-being, and ecstasy.

In this book, an essay is made on the sound phenomena and its use as a therapeutic procedure. Starting with a brief passage on the History of Music since antiquity until the early 20th century, the text proceeds with a description of the nature of sound waves and the behavior of vibrating systems, such as strings, tubes, and membranes.

The content has no technical character, and the intention is to provide an easy-to-read topic for anyone with some curiosity about this subject. Next, the nature and formation of a musical scale are discussed, drawing attention to the mathematical basis of the formation of musical intervals.

The mechanism of hearing is then presented to provide a short description of the structure of the human auditory system as well as to highlight the range of our perception of the sound waves within the audible interval. Acoustics is a branch of science of crucial importance in describing the distribution and propagation of sound in an ambient as well as in resonant cavities. A short description is presented about important and fundamental aspects of the acoustic design of a room.

In ancient Greece, *Psykhe* was the goddess of the soul and wife of Eros, the god of love. Today, psyche means the soul, mind, spirit, or invisible animating entity which occupies the physical body. The feelings, thoughts, and perceptions developed by our psyche determine our adaptation to the ambiance in which we live and to which we relate throughout processes of a very particular character, the result of our life experiences and perceptions of the world. The unconscious and music can be related from the perspective of analytical psychology, where it can be seen as a stimulus to the transcendence of consciousness, favoring the evocation of images from the psyche.

In brief, the psyche and music correlation is approached to emphasize its capacity as a form of expression to reduce the ego's defenses and to induce relaxation, thereby helping in the transition to an altered state of consciousness, which may contribute to enhance the positive outcomes of treatment strategies of a therapeutic process.

Music therapy is addressed here in the spotlight. This is, by definition, the clinical and evidence-based use of musical interventions to achieve individualized goals, within a therapeutic relation directed by an accredited professional. It is the use of music to improve people's quality of life. In dealing with emotions and feelings, the possibilities of their good use have found increasing recognition worldwide among health professionals.

With the advancement of knowledge about the functioning of our brain, music therapy is gaining more and more importance for the achievement of emotional balance and well-being. In a music therapy procedure the sonorous stimulus assimilated by the patient submitted to the treatment is transformed into particular sensations and emotions, for a beneficial and quite positive effect.

Acoustic vibrational therapies are then discussed from the concepts of physics. In a broader sense, in addition to traditional music therapy, these also include procedures with diverse stimuli such as ultrasound therapy, which have been successfully applied in a variety of applications in healing procedures.

Sound therapy then refers to all proposals for treatment conveyed by the application of acoustic signals to any living organisms (humans, animals, and plants) to promote good health, to stimulate healthy development or even as a complementary procedure of cure.

In this sense is the concept of the Mozart effect, introduced in 1991 by the French researcher Alfred A. Tomatis, who believed that polyphonic music could promote the cure of a variety of diseases as well as contributes to brain development.

From then on, several reports appeared on the use of music pointing out beneficial results in plants and animals. Farmers have bet on the use of a musical background to improve the cultivation of plants, to stimulate milk production of cows and even for the production of bananas and grapes.

With the growing technological revolution we see today, and the scientific advance in the most varied areas of knowledge such as neuroscience, physics, chemistry and biology, we can imagine that in the very near future we will enjoy much more sophisticated vibrational therapies than the ones we have today, aimed at promoting healing by speeding up a health recovery treatment as well as providing better quality of life and greater well-being for everyone.

There is, obviously, a long way to go in order to consolidate new studies and develop experimental researches that may enable the discovery of new therapeutic procedures with scientifically proven efficacy.

At last but not least, we provide a digression on the fascinating topic of Celestial Music. This was born from the harmonic concept of *Music of the Spheres* of the ancient Greeks, which incorporated the Pythagorean view that mathematical relations express harmonies that manifest themselves in numbers and sounds with a singular pattern of proportion. This remained for a long time as a paradigm of harmony and a reflex of the stability of the cosmic order and of the perfection of the divine creation.

The standards of harmony and aesthetics in the past sought to reflect the celestial harmony for the preservation of good order and social equilibrium. The concepts of beauty and perfection therefore relied on the harmony of forms and balance of proportions, which spread widely in all creative expressions in all kinds of arts.

Spiritualists also speak about the existence of a sublime *heavenly melody*, present in all creation, and unequaled with *earthly melody*. Following the law of affinity, we attract what we think or feel, and so our spirit must vibrate according to the stimuli received.

Music has the capacity to be used as an important auxiliary support of a therapeutic process, in which it can contribute positively in a variety of treatments, such as post-operative recovery, post-traumatic, behavior disorders, or even in a psychoanalytic context to facilitate the expression of the subject by allowing emotional associations and sublimation of unconscious drives.

When listening to pleasant music there is a neurochemical alteration with a discharge of dopamine in the listener. This is a powerful neurotransmitter that plays a key role in the induction and maintenance of essential activities needed to maintain a healthy body, such as food consumption and sex, among others, and which is also responsible for the different patterns of drug addiction behavior.

Good motivational music contributes to the elevation of the spirit, and the more developed the sensitivity of the listener, the more relish one can enjoy. The sense of overjoy, rapture, and delight we can experience allows us to be more predisposed to good influences and suggestible to more positive feelings. The sublime music is like a prayer that gives us enchantment and contributes to the elevation of our innermost feelings.

1. Brief History of Music

In the history of mankind we can imagine that the earliest musical manifestations probably were born from intonations applied to cries, howls and whistles, loaded with feelings, accompanied by beats and strokes following a rhythm, created at a moment of celebration and collective euphoria. The verbal expression of strong emotions of the primitive man, as in a painful lament or by expressing great jubilation after a successful accomplishment, could follow the intonation of a ditty, and thus the vocalization reinforced by the musical inflection became a song.

It is interesting to wonder what would have been the first musical instrument created by the primitive man to produce sequential sounds, in a controlled way. Probably this could have been an object of percussion, which produced different types of sound from beating in other objects, like stones, trunks, bones, etc.

Among the first instruments used by our ancestors in prehistory must surely be also some kind of whistle, the precursor of the flute. A few years ago scientists discovered artifacts made from bird bones and mammoth ivory in caves on the slopes of mountains in southwestern

Germany, which, according to some, are the oldest musical instruments ever found in the world, dating to about 40000 years old. This coincides with the period when the first anatomically modern humans were spreading through Central Europe, along the Danube River valley, before the last ice age.

The evolution of the musical instruments naturally accompanied the technological development of primitive societies, upon handling different materials. With the mastery of metal technologies even more sophisticated wind instruments were being produced.

The origin of musical creation is lost in time and is directly linked to the ability to produce more elaborated sounds rhythmically, either by voice modulation or via the use of instruments of varied sonority. With the advent of the writing came also the possibility of definitively recording songs and melodies. Cave paintings dating back to about 15000 years illustrate dance scenes that were probably accompanied by chants following some rhythm.

While the earliest writing records are dated to about 5000 BC, those identified as truly musical are from an ancient song found in cuneiform writing, dated 4000 BC, discovered in the city of Ur, ancient Mesopotamia, now Iraq. This was composed in harmonic intervals of the third, using a diatonic scale, which was recognized until very recently as an exclusive characteristic of the Western music.[1]

This finding then identifies the time of the beginning of the civilized ancient music, that is, of that present in cultures that have made written records. Fragments of papyrus from ancient Egypt containing a kind of musical notation of a song were found, with indications that vocal art had a prominent position in the society at that time.

Although cultures from the East have had their musical evolution occurring independently, the records available in the Western Academy are almost exclusively from the Occidental culture. It is interesting to note that the term ancient music refers not only to that of ancient Sumerian, Egyptian, Greek, Roman, Renaissance, Baroque, Asian, Muslim but also to a musical style still performed today.

However, whatever the first form of musical manifestation of humankind, it certainly arised from the intimate desire to express a feeling to establish a communication of the inner self with the surroundings, such as to express deep joy or sadness, in moments of celebration or revolt.

---

[1] Steven Mithen. The Singing Neanderthals: The Origins of Music, Language, Mind, and Body. Harvard University Press, Oct 2007.

In this sense, anyone can create some kind of melody to express an intimate feeling. In the presence of others, this is also a way to communicate and to share feelings. Music is then a direct mode of instantaneous connection between our soul and the universe.

Little is known of the musical instruments used in antiquity beyond the meager traces that have come to these days. Most of that we know today have been identified in frescoes, murals, and paintings.

A bas-relief from the time of Assurbanipal (705-681 BC), king of Assyria, shows a parade where one can identify lira players with seven strings.[2] In 1929 Leonard Woolley discovered fragments of three harps in the ruins of the ancient city of Ur, formerly Mesopotamia, now guarded, part in the Penn Museum, the Museum of Archaeology and Anthropology of the University of Pennsylvania (USA), and part in the British Museum in London.

The earliest records that have been found dealing with the creation and analysis of a musical scale are due to Pythagoras, a Greek philosopher, and mathematician who was born on the island of Samos, between about 571 BC and 570 BC, and died in Metapontum around 496 BC.

---

[2] Bozhidar Abrahev. Illustrated Encyclopedia of Musical Instruments. Konemann, Oct 2000.

Pythagoras considered the father of musical theory, founded a mystical and philosophical school that regarded numbers as the essence, the fundamental principles that form all things. The symbol of this school was the pentagram, the five-pointed star. For the Pythagoreans there existed four primordial elements: earth, water, fire, and air.

The word music derives from the Greek *mousike*, referring to the art of the nine muses: *Clio, Euterpe, Thalia, Melpomeni, Terpsichore, Erato, Polymnia, Ourania, and Calliope.* [3] These were deities that give artists and philosophers the inspiration for creation in all kinds of artistic manifestations. The word *mousike* then referred to everything that was intended for the exercise of the mind, including mathematics. Plato used to say that musical training, combined with gymnastics, is the most powerful instrument for the benefit of the soul.

The culture of the body in ancient Greece was based on the concept that the soul deserves a temple worthy of its occupation, and the combination of gymnastics and music produces a harmonious balance between soul and body. Music awakens admiration for beauty and balance, bringing mental and moral discipline, while gymnastics brings physical strength and courage (*Mens Sana in Corpore Sano*).

---

[3] B.V.M. de Sá. História da música. Casa Moreira de Sá, 1920.

Practically nothing came to us from the music of ancient Greece and Rome. In the remnants and fragments found concerning art, there is nothing about musical notation. It is known however that Homer's epic poems and Sappho's lyrics were sung with instrumental accompaniment, but there are no records about his metric and punctuation.

Fragments of Greek music were found in the choral work of Euripides and some hymns of Mesomedes of Crete (2nd century AD). Until very recently it was believed that the music of antiquity was purely monophonic and that polyphony was then an invention of the Middle Ages. However, archaeological shreds of evidence of new findings contradict this point of view. A musical record dated about 4000 years was deciphered by Prof. Anne D. Kilmer of the University of California at Berkeley. This is composed of a harmony that uses intervals of thirds and a diatonic scale.

Therefore, not even the diatonic scale can be considered a Western creation. The double tubes used by the Greeks in old flutes and pipes, as seen in illustrations on ancient vases and walls, demonstrate that there was also notions of harmony with chords at that time.

The Badarian culture, which developed between 4400-4000 BC in el-Badari, at Upper Egypt and the Eastern Desert, provided the earliest evidence of agriculture in ancient Egypt where a considerable advance is observed. About forty settlements and six hundred tombs were located, and records of social stratification were identified from the burial of the more prosperous members of the community.

The Badarian economy was mainly based on agriculture, fishing, and livestock. Their tools included scrapers, drills, axes, bifacial scythes, and concave-base arrowheads, and their main crops included wheat, barley, lentils, and tubers. The Badarians were the ancestors of the ancient Egyptians and were a mixture of races. The excavations showed fragments of a type of harp, a chordophone, which has its strings positioned perpendicular to the resonant body.

The oldest stringed instrument that has been found is an Egyptian harp, identified from drawings of a mural of the fourth dynasty, dated to about 3000 BC. This was a simple triangular instrument with a bow, developed from the hunting bow. It used to have from eight to twelve strings and was played by the musician sitting, standing or kneeling. These were usually made of wood.

Ancient Egyptian music was based on a smaller pentatonic scale of five full tones, with no semitones. This was deduced from the positions of holes in flutes. During the New Empire, wars and conquests by foreigners put the Egyptians in closer contact with the Asian peoples and their musical culture, and therefore many new instruments were created, and with them, new sound qualities were introduced.

The most popular string instrument in ancient Greece was the lyre, considered as the symbol of the god Apollo. From the remnants of some old instruments recently found in Iraq, which appear to be lyres or harps, several reconstructions were attempted, but none were considered satisfactory. The most famous is a bull-headed harp, and several attempts are still being made to build a replica of it to be part of an orchestra destined to the local tourism.

Harps are also identified in murals from the time of Ramesses III of Egypt, dating from about 1200 BC. Several types of ancient harps were found in Africa, Europe, North, and South America, as well as in parts of Asia. The earliest documented references are from 4000 BC in Egypt up to about 3000 BC in Mesopotamia. This is also mentioned in most Bible translations, and King David was the most prominent harpist at that time. A sort of tuner was introduced in the second half of the 17th century to allow changes in the tuning of a string by a semitone.

The European harp appears to have originated in Ireland about a thousand years ago. In Irish mythology, a magic species was mentioned. In South America and Mexico there are also ancient models, which seem to be derived from the baroque harps brought from Spain during the colonial period. The Paraguayan is the most popular, and it is currently the national instrument of the country. It has about 36 strings with narrow spacing and lighter tension than the more traditional ones and thus has a slightly more grave pitch.

Egyptian music evolved as a rich blend of Indian, Arab, African and Western influences. Ancient records show that in about 4000 BC the Egyptians were already playing harps and flutes, as well as two-stringed instruments of indigenous origin, *ney*, and *oud*. However, no complete record of musical composition was found until the 7th century AD, when Egypt became part of the Arab world. It is known, however, that percussion and singing were already important at that time. Belly dancing seems to have originated in ancient Egypt, and today the country is considered the center of reference for this art.

Egyptian musical instruments were reasonably well developed and varied. Among the various types identified in ancient paintings and murals, we can see stringed instruments such as harps, lyres, lutes, and percussion instruments such as drums, rattles, tambourines, bells, cymbals, as well as wind instruments such as flutes and trumpets.

The flutes are among the musical instruments most used in antiquity. Double flutes were known from about

2800 BC, constructed of two parallel tubes, which were later separated and adjusted at an acute angle. These are still used in Egypt these days. In the 2nd century BC in ancient Rome was invented a sort of hydraulic organ, which used water pressure to supply air to sound pipes.

In ancient music, the principal instruments used were the harp, the lyre, the flute, the trumpet, the oboe, and the organ. In the Middle Ages among the main instruments were the organ and the lute. The former was an instrument still primitive at that time, whose keys were operated by a blow with the fist. The lute is a stringed instrument with an arm with frets and a rounded bulge. This evolved from an instrument originally used in ancient Persia, now Iran called *barbat*, which is also the ancestor of *oud*, something similar, and used in ancient Egypt. The words *lute* and *oud* are both derived from Arabic *al'ud*, meaning wood.

The lute player is called a lutenist and the lute maker is called a luthier. Lutes are made almost exclusively of wood. The front of the instrument is a thin flat blade of wood as in a classical guitar, whereas in the back it has a bulge with oval shape, like gout. Usually, these have a single hole under the ropes, called a rosette; and some more elaborate show several rosettes. The hole is not open like in the acoustic guitar but covered with a thin grid of wood in the shape of a vine entwined, carved directly into the top wood.

The back is mounted from thin strips of wood called ribs, in the form of strips like banana peels, attached at the tip to form a rounded body for the instrument. In the baroque era, the body was turned back to better hold the ropes and maintains the tuning. It is very difficult to tune this instrument in its old version.

In medieval times the first records of polyphonic music appeared in France, mainly from the 11th century, but these still represented a basic notation without an accurate designation of tones.

In the formation of European society during the Dark Ages, between the disintegration of the Roman Empire and the predominance of the Catholic Church, dozens of mini-kingdoms were established, each ruled by a feudal lord. These, in turn, lived under the strong influence of powerful Catholic leaders.

The Church was thus able to dictate the progress of the arts and letters according to their restrictions, and Western music was the practically exclusive property of the Catholic Church. The so-called Dark Ages comprise most of the Middle Ages, in a period which extends to about 6 to 13 centuries, and designates an era that goes as far as the rise of the Italian Renaissance in the 14th century.

Gregorian chant designates a monophonic vocal genre that comprises a single melody, without any harmonic support or accompaniment, with a flexible rhythm, without metric, adapted by the Benedictine monk Gregory I (540-604 AD), a pope of the Catholic Church, to be used in the religious celebrations.

This was the official musical practice of the Roman Catholic Church for more than 1000 years. The text was the essence of the Gregorian chant. From this proceed the Gregorian modes major (Ionian) and minor (Aeolian), in addition to five less known modes: Doric, Phrygian, Lithium, Mixolydian, and Locrian. Before the 6th century, one cannot speak of Gregorian chant, and the general denomination for the melodies sung at that time would, therefore, be simply religious singing.

The chant is the denomination applied to the monophonic practice of singing used in Christian liturgies, but of pagan origin. Arising in the nuclei of the Church in Constantinople, Rome, Antioch, and Jerusalem chanting designate the various forms of Christian rites such as the Ambrosian, Gregorian, Galician, Ancient Roman and Mozarabic. Formed mainly by intervals of seconds and thirds, the chant is the basis of Western ancient music.

In the medieval (or Gothic) period, which lies approximately between 800-1400 AD, the songs were an integral part of everyday life, especially during festivities and celebrations events. Among the most common instruments were horns, whistles, bells, and drums. It was also quite common to play cheerful and lively music during meals because it was believed at that time that this was not only pleasing to hearing but also aided in the digestion of food.

Many musical traditions of the West can be traced back to the social and religious developments that occurred in Europe during the Middle Ages, particularly between 500 and 1300 AD. Due to the strong domination of the Catholic Church in this period, sacred music was predominant. Beginning with the Gregorian chant, it developed slowly into a more polyphonic version, originally called *organum*, which was performed in the French cathedrals in the tube and bellows organs of the 12th century.

Medieval music flourished among the French troubadours until it culminated in the sacred and secular compositions of the French composer and poet Guillaume de Machaut (1300-1377), recognized as the greatest genius composer of the western world of that time, and principal exponent of the so-called *ars nova*, polyphonic music of the 14th century.

Musical notation transformed the work of several Christian priests, especially the monk Guido D'Arezzo (992-1050 AD), the main responsible for the adoption of the line system, from which the current musical pattern originated. It is him who designated the musical notes as they are known today, using the text of a Latin hymn to St. John the Baptist, where each phrase begins in a musical tone: *Ut queant laxis, Resonare fibris, Mira gestorum, Famuli tuorum, Solve polluti, Labii reatum, Sancte Ioannes*, which means "That thy servants may be able to resound clearly the wonder of thy deeds, cleanse our unclean lips, O St. John." Thus, the initial syllable of each verse was taken as the name for the musical note corresponding to that tone.

Earlier the notes were designated by the first seven letters of the Latin alphabet. In this way, the musical notes came to be called UT, RE, MI, FA, SOL, LA and SI. Subsequently, the name DO replace the UT. The name of the note SI was formed from the initial letters of the last verse of the hymn, *Sancte Ioannes*.

In the East, music has always been an important part of the life of the Indian people, ranging from simple melodies to the most developed classical themes. There are references to various types of string and wind instruments, and various types of drums and plates in the Vedas. Muslim rulers and nobles supported the musical demonstrations and kept their patronage to the musicians.

Hindustani and Carnatic are traditions of Indian classical music, originated in the north and south of the country, respectively, around the thirteenth and fourteenth centuries. The first was influenced not only by the older traditions and the Vedic philosophy but also by Persian elements.

Carnatic has a rich history and is one of the jewels of world culture. Since the 16th century, the division between Indian music from the north and south regions became more clearly delineated. Both can be instrumental or vocal. The zither is one of the most popular instruments in northern India. This has a long neck with twenty metal frets and six to seven main ropes, where a gourd acts as a resonator.

Indian classical music is based on ragas, which are the scales and melodies that provide the basis of an execution. Unlike the West, Indian allows for a much greater degree of customization of performance, almost at the level of jazzist improvisation. Each performance of a raga is different, and its purpose is to create a state of trance.

The Indian ragas were created over the centuries in a continuous evolutionary process and sought to reflect a more universal view of the world without the connotation of individual emotions. Many ragas share the same scale or the same melodic theme. Although there are thousands of ragas, only six are considered fundamental: *Bhairav, Malkauns, Hindel, Dipak, Megh, and Shree.*

Popular music also existed during the Middle Ages, unrelated to the traditions of the Church. It did not even have written records, but hundreds of these songs were later recorded by bands of flourishing musicians throughout Europe, especially from the 12th century, by French troubadours. They were usually monophonic melodies with improvised accompaniment, and rhythmically well animated, whose main theme was love. One of the most famous composers of this time is Adam de la Halle (1237-1286 AD).

In the Middle Ages, the period of European history that lies between about 450-1450 AD, there were two important artistic periods: the Romanesque (1000-1150) and the Gothic (1150-1450). The most important musicians of that time were mainly priests and monks. During the Middle Ages, the women were not allowed to enter the church.

A woman was, however, an important composer of that time: Hildegard of Bingen (1098-1179), who left a legacy of a large number of compositions which survived the time. She was a German Benedictine nun, mystic, theologian, composer, preacher, naturalist, medical doctor, poetess, playwright, writer, and mistress of the Rupertsberg

Monastery in Bingen am Rhein, Germany. [4] It was proclaimed Doctor of the Universal Church, by Pope Benedict XVI, in an apostolic letter of October 7, 2012.

The era of Renaissance music encompasses the period between the medieval and the baroque, i.e., the early 15th and early 17th centuries. Several important instruments emerged at this time, such as the harpsichord, the psaltery (a mechanized form of a stringed instrument fingering), the spinet and the violin family.

The term Renaissance is relatively recent. In his *Histoire de France*, the French philosopher and historian Jules Michelet (1798-1874) coined this word to designate the period from about 1450-1600, known as the *Quattrocento* (1400) and *Cinquecento* (1500).

The term *Humanism* goes hand in hand with Renaissance and places a new emphasis on the human rather than the spiritual. The designation of *Renaissance Humanism* originated in the 13th century, is used to differentiate it from the *Humanism* that came later. The idea of humanism also implied the revival of ancient Greek culture that influenced the arts in general. It is also associated with classicism, that is, the classical understanding of form, balance, and symmetry.

---

[4] Hildegard Von Bingen's Physica: The Complete English Translation of Her Classic Work on Health and Healing 31 ago 1998 by Hildegard of Bingen (Author), Priscilla Throop (Editor).

Around 1450 Johann Gutenberg developed the press in Europe based on the Chinese movable type of print. Therefore, in the year 1473, the first editions of liturgical books were published on Gregorian singing.

The term baroque was first used in the mid-18th century. The word comes from the Portuguese *Barocco*, which means a deformed pearl. The term later assumed a negative connotation, indicating something bizarre, exaggerated, and grotesque, even in bad taste. The term was rescued by musicologists to mean about a century and a half of the history of European music (1600-1750).

The Baroque period was also simultaneous with that of the Enlightenment (*Illuminism*), during which the sciences, the arts, and literature had great production, with new inventions and scientific discoveries.

It was particularly in the Baroque period when the first musical orchestras were formed, which was responsible for the first operas, a complex and thematic musical works, accompanied by staging and artistic characterization.

As the Church of that time forbade the execution of operas in their domains, a new style of composition appeared, the *Oratorium*, which did not differ much from the structure of the opera but was directed to a religious theme. Since then, new musical styles have emerged:

Cantata, Concerto Grosso, Trio, Sonata, Suite, Fugue, among others.

Amid the great composers of this period are John Dowland (1563-1626), Tomaso Albinoni (1671-1750), Antonio Lucio Vivaldi (1678-1741), Georg Philipp Telemann (1681-1767), George Frideric Handel (1685-1759) and Johann Sebastian Bach (1685-1750).

Pre-Classicism refers to that period in the history of music-making the transition between baroque and classicism, having its greatest exponents in the Neapolitan opera. Further on is the classicism (1750-1820), where the sonata becomes the most important musical form of the late 18th and early 19th centuries.

This initially designated a polyphonic piece, instrumental, in opposition to the symphony, which is more homophonic. Later on, came the *sonata*, in *fugue* style, and the *chamber sonata*, composed of a suite of dances. From this time are Wilhelm Friedemann Bach (1710-1784), Carl Philipp Emanuel Bach (1714-1788), Franz Joseph Haydn (1732-1806), Wolfgang Amadeus Mozart (1756-1791), Ludwig Van Beethoven (1770-1827), Niccolo Paganini (1782-1840), Carl Maria von Weber (1786-1826), Gioachino Antonio Rossini (1792-1868) and Franz Peter Schubert (1797-1828).

In Brazil of that period lived José Joaquim Emérico Lobo de Mesquita (1746-1805), composer, teacher, conductor and organist, Manuel Dias de Oliveira (1734-1813), and José Maurício Nunes Garcia (1767-1830), this latter being one of the greatest exponents of Classicism in the Americas.[5]

Romanticism refers to the period 1830-1900, when music was more emotional and more expressive, whose emphasis was more important than the formal or structural considerations of the Classical era. The Classical period is generally used to refer to the post-Baroque and Pre-Romantic eras, between 1750 and 1830, and covers the development of classical symphony and concert.

It was an orderly, well-balanced composition with qualities of clarity and balance, formally perfected, emphasizing formal rather than emotional beauty. The Classical period is sometimes also called *rococo*. From that time came the development of the orchestra and large musical forms, especially the symphony. It was the time of, among many, Louis-Hector Berlioz (1803-1869), Johann Strauss I (1804-1849), Jacob Ludwig Felix Mendelssohn (1809-1847), Frederic Chopin (1810-1849), Robert Alexander Schumann (1810 -1856), Franz Liszt

---

[5] An interesting description of the Brazilian music:
http://www.gazetadebeirute.com/2012/12/historia-da-musica-brasil
eira.html

(1811-1886), Wilhelm Richard Wagner (1813-1883), Giuseppe Fortunino Frencesco Verdi (1813-1901) and Peter Ilyich Tchaikovsky (1840-1893).

Impressionism (1880-1920) emerged in France in the mid-19th century as a new way of perceiving the world, especially in music and the plastic arts, with the appreciation of the sonority of musical instruments and harmonic games. Among the exponents of that time are Claude Debussy (1862-1918) and Maurice Ravel (1875-1937).

With the manifestation of the rebellious art of modernity began the so-called Modernism (1910-1940), characterized by rhythmic research, the use of various shades (polytonalism) or none (atonalism). Great composers of this age are Heitor Villa-Lobos (1887-1959), Arnold Schoenberg (1874-1951), Igor Stravinsky (1882-1971), George Gershwin (1898-1937), Duke Ellington (1899-1974), Dmitri Shostakovich -1975), John Cage (1912-1992), Benjamin Britten (1913-1976), Leonard Bernstein (1918-1990). From there begins the period of contemporary music.[6]

---

[6] It is important to emphasize that is far the pretension of exhausting herein the list of names of the eminent composers of the past. The mention of a few is just fortuitous and occasional. A vast literature can be easily found on this subject.

The musical heritage of the humankind connects us all in this planet as a single race, united by our moral and sentimental identity via the deepest channels of our inner humanity.

2. Waves and Vibrating Systems

Sound is an undulatory phenomenon that propagates through longitudinal mechanical waves, i.e., an oscillatory motion where the vibration of the medium occurs along the direction of propagation of the wave. Thus, in the vacuum, it is not possible to propagate the sound. From a microscopic point of view, we can consider a plane wavefront to visualize the shifting of the air molecules with the passage of a sound wave.

The displacement of the surface of a plane wavefront causes a compression of the layer of air immediately adjacent, thereby causing a local increase in air density in the form of a compression pulse. This push, in turn, creates a zone of adjacent rarefaction behind, and thus, for each pulse of compression there is a zone of rarefaction that accompanies it, and then begins a periodic movement that propagates as a longitudinal wave.

The speed of propagation of sound waves in a medium depends very much on their characteristics. The elastic properties of the medium have a great influence on how these waves are transmitted and attenuated during the crossing. In the air, for example, the speed of sound is about 343 m/s. However, air temperature and humidity also affect the velocity of propagation. In freshwater, the speed of sound is 1493 m/s, in seawater, 1533 m/s, in iron 5130 m/s and diamond, 12000 m/s.

The study of modes of sound propagation and the way it disperses in a medium represents a vast field of study within the scope of acoustics. The sources of sound waves can vary widely, since almost every natural event that occurs in nature, whether on the surface of the Earth, in the atmosphere or even in the interior of the planet, produces sound. In musical instruments, the sound waves are produced by vibrating strings, sound tubes, and vibrating membranes.

Among the various types of wave are the following categories:

- Mechanical waves

- Electromagnetic waves

- Matter waves

Mechanical waves are those that propagate only in material media, such as waves in water, waves in a rope, seismic waves and sound waves. Electromagnetic waves otherwise do not need a medium for propagation and are generated by oscillating electric and magnetic fields. These cover a wide range of frequencies, the so-called electromagnetic spectrum, which includes AM and FM radio waves, TV waves, X-rays, gamma rays and cosmic rays. Matter waves are those described by quantum mechanics to represent any moving particle, the so-called *de Broglie* waves.

While in a longitudinal wave the vibration of the medium occurs in the same direction of propagation, in the transverse waves the vibration is perpendicular to the direction of propagation. Among the latter are the waves on a rope and the electromagnetic waves. The amplitude of a mechanical wave is the measure of the maximum displacement of a point in the medium where the wave propagates, taken from the equilibrium position (zero displacement).

The wavelength λ is the distance between two points in which the waveform repeats, for example, between two crests (points of maximum amplitude). The speed at which a wave propagates is given by velocity = distance/time. It is written, $v = \lambda/T$, where T represents the wave period, i.e., the repetition time, which is the time interval corresponding to a complete vibration.

The frequency f of the wave is the number of oscillations per second, which is equal to the inverse of the period, i.e., $f = 1/T$, and is given in Hertz (Hz). Thus we have $\lambda \times f = v$. The velocity of a mechanical wave also depends on the elastic properties of the medium where it propagates, such as volumetric compressibility and specific mass.

The intensity of a wave is a measure of the power (energy/time) of the wave by the area it hits ($I=P/A$). In common language when we refer to the "height" of a perceived sound, we mean the sound level, the term scientifically correct. This uses a logarithmic scale, more appropriate to sweep a large range of values, measured in decibels (dB). The threshold of human hearing is 0 dB, a rustle of leaves is about 10 dB, a normal conversation, 60 dB, and the pain threshold, 120 dB. However, prolonged exposure to sounds above 100 dB can cause definitive hearing loss.

When two sounds are produced with close frequencies, the sound we heard which results from their combination has oscillating intensity, called a beat. The frequency we heard is given by their average frequency. For example, if sound waves of 340 Hz and 350 Hz are produced simultaneously, a person would hear a sound of 345 Hz, varying in intensity (amplitude) 10 times per second. The combined sound is then heard at a frequency slightly different from that of the original sounds with an intensity that oscillates with a frequency given by the difference of their frequencies.

This is used by instrument tuners to adjust the sound of vibrating strings or sound tubes to produce the precisely correct note. In the strings, we adjust the tension, whereas, in the tubes, we adjust the length by adding or removing small pieces to fit the tube to the appropriate size.

When the source of sound waves is moving relatively to the listener, the sound perceived has a peculiar effect, called the Doppler Effect. This is what happens, for example, in a car race where one hears a change in the tone when the car is approaching or when it is moving away.

The sonic Doppler Effect is then the change in the frequency heard when there is a relative movement between source and listener. It was first analyzed by the Austrian J.C. Doppler in 1842. But this occurs not only for sound waves but also for electromagnetic waves. When both the source and observer approach each other, an increase in the frequency occurs. If they move away relatively to each other, there is a reduction in the observed frequency.

The most common musical instruments can be classified as of wind, string or percussion instruments. These comprise sound tubes with resonant air columns, vibrating strings fixed on appropriate supports for adjustment of tension, or stretched and tensioned skins or sheets, composing vibrating surfaces, or even objects that produce sounds utilizing strokes, friction, shaking, etc.

The instruments found belonging to the earliest civilizations represent the most varied artifacts used to produce sounds using beats and strokes in wood, gourds, resonant boxes made of bone or wood, whistles, and flutes, in an immense variety of forms and arrangements. In these, the vibrating object places the surrounding air in vibration at the same frequency, and this movement propagates as a progressive sound wave that travels and is attenuated as it moves away from the source.

When two waves traveling in opposite directions meet, the effect from their superposition and combination can generate the phenomenon of interference. Depending on how this superposition occurs, the observed effect may be of magnification (or reinforcement) of the undulating phenomenon or even its cancellation.

In the first case, we have constructive interference, and in the second case, destructive interference. However, upon interfering, the waves act independently and may even resume their original form after interfering. For example, if two pulses on a string traveling in opposite directions meet at a certain region, there will be an overlap at the rendezvous point, but these will continue to propagate independently of each other after the encounter, without losing the original shape.

A particularly important effect is the formation of standing waves, which are the basis of the sound emission of musical instruments. When an isolated pulse propagates on a long, stretched rope, each point changes its position as the ripple passes. Thus, this point leaves its equilibrium position, reaches maximum displacement, until it returns to rest once the pulse has passed. This happens in a very short time.

When a stretched string attached to the ends (like in a guitar for example) is put to vibrate by fingering, the ends remain attached and constitute nodes or points of zero amplitude. Standing waves are then produced by the interference of the reflected waves in the extremities of the rope. Thus, there are points on the vibrating string which have null displacement (nodes) or maximum displacement (antinodes).

Unlike the progressive wave, which travels on a rope that has only one end attached, in the standing wave the amplitude of vibration of each point of the rope depends on its position. The nodes and antinodes occur in specific and well-defined positions. Thus we have the formation of the so-called harmonic modes of standing waves on a vibrating string attached at both ends.

Each oscillation mode represents a natural resonant vibration frequency of the stretched string. The reflected waves at the fixed ends overlap constructively. Thus, the first mode of oscillation also called the fundamental mode (or first harmonic), is that in which the string vibrates at a frequency where the length L is equal to half the wavelength λ, i.e., $L = \lambda/2$.

The second harmonic corresponds to that mode of vibration where $L = 2\,\lambda/2 = \lambda$. The third harmonic is obtained from $L = 3\,\lambda/2$, and so on. Therefore, the so-called harmonic series corresponding to the modes of vibration of standing waves produced in a stretched rope with fixed extremities is obtained from $n\,\lambda/2 = L$, where $n = 1,2,3 \ldots$

The sound produced by a vibrating string also depends on its mass, in addition to the tension. Thicker strings vibrate more slowly, have lower frequencies, and the longer and thicker the string, the more grave is the emitted sound.

To vibrate, the string may be fingered, played with a pick or a bow. For a wave on a stretched string, the propagation velocity is determined by the specific mass and the tensile force (T) to which the rope is subjected and which keeps it strained. The specific mass (M) is the mass of the rope divided by its linear length, which indicates the amount of matter per unit length. Hence, the velocity of a wave in the string is given by $v = (T/m)^{1/2}$.

The oldest stringed instrument found is an Egyptian harp, identified from drawings of a mural from the fourth dynasty, dated to about 3000 BC. This was a simple triangular instrument with a bow. The most popular string instrument in ancient Greece was the lyre, considered as the symbol of the god Apollo. On a guitar, the string is strummed, vibrating the bridge, which then vibrates the top and the air in the inner cavity, as well as the back and sides. The guitar body then acts to cause the vibrations of the bridge to be transformed into low-pressure vibrations of the surrounding air.

When a sound wave propagates in the air the molecules move back and forth in the oscillatory motion, and the local pressure of the air also varies in an oscillating way by very small quantities. The number of vibrations per second is the frequency, measured in cycles per second (Hz).

The tone of a musical note is determined by its frequency: high pitch has high frequency and low pitch means low frequency. For example, the tone A corresponding to the fifth string of the guitar has a frequency of 440 Hz. The loose strings of the guitar have the frequencies: 329.64 Hz (E), 440 Hz (A), 587.33 Hz (D), 783.99 Hz (G), 987.77 Hz (B), and 1318.51 Hz (E).

The body of a musical instrument contributes to transmit the vibrations to the surrounding air. For this, it needs, therefore, a large surface area, to vibrate a large quantity of air. On a guitar, for example, the top is made to vibrate up and down relatively easily. The backplate is much less important for most frequencies because it is against the body of the musician. The sides do not vibrate in the direction perpendicular to its surface and thus radiate less.

However, the air inside the body of the musical instrument plays a very important role in its acoustics performance, especially at low frequencies. It vibrates similarly to the air trapped in a bottle when one blows near the nozzle. If one plays a note between F# and A, keeping the ear close to the hole in the guitar top, he can hear the air inside resonates.

The frequencies of the resonance modes generally do not follow a simple harmonic progression. For example, the frequency of the first harmonic for a single vibrating string is twice that of the fundamental mode, whereas for a vibrating surface this is not twice the frequency of that one.

Keyboard instruments are those in which sounds are produced by the action of keys. These operate as a lever, and when its outer end is touched, it is lowered, while the other end immediately rises and triggers the mechanism that produces the sound, for example, by vibrating a string inside the instrument. There are different types of mechanisms that originate the sounds by keys, so there are also different types of instruments, such as the piano, the harpsichord, and the organ, among others.

The first keyboards appeared in the 3rd century BC, when Ctesibios of Alexandria, an engineer from ancient Greece, invented an organ that was an instrument that consisted of a water box, where there was a manually operated air pump, and a large keyboard that controlled the air outlet through 8 to 10 tubes. The keys were not touched with the fingers but struck with the fists. The black keys gradually emerged from the 12th century, and only at the beginning of the 15th century that the keyboard was made as we know it today.

When the air vibrates inside a hollow tube, opened at the ends, regions of condensation (high pressure) and rarefaction (low pressure) are produced inside, which propagate in the form of sound waves. If the frequency of these waves is such that their wavelength equals the length of the tube, the superposition of the waves propagating in opposite directions produces a standing wave pattern corresponding to the harmonic. Such frequencies are the so-called resonant frequencies of the tube.

The waves which emerge at each end of the tube then have the same frequency of the air vibrations inside the tube. Each end behaves like an antinode, that is, a region where the air vibrates with the largest amplitude. If one end of the tube is closed, then there will be formed a node, i.e., a region where the vibration amplitude of the air is zero.

The possible resonant frequencies to be excited in a tube of length L with both ends opened thus correspond to the harmonic series $L = n\,\lambda/2$, where $n = 1,2,3...$, is the harmonic number. As in a string, the fundamental mode or first harmonic corresponds to $n = 1$. Recalling that $\lambda \times f = v$, then we have for the frequencies of the harmonic series $f = v/\lambda = nv/2L$.

In a tube with only one end opened, the simpler standing wave pattern requires the condition that the wavelength inside the tube is such that $L = \lambda/4$. This oscillation mode corresponds to the largest standing wavelength that can be generated in the tube, or equivalently, the lowest frequency. The next value of λ which produces a standing wave is given by $L = 3\lambda/4$, and so on. The harmonic series of the standing wave frequencies in a tube with only one open end is then obtained from $L = n\,\lambda/4$, where $n = 1,3,5...$ (n odd).

It is important to note that the length of an instrument, whether of vibrating strings or tubes with vibrating air columns, defines a range of operation for the production of harmonic frequencies. Larger instruments are intended to produce a standing wave pattern corresponding to oscillation modes defined by larger wavelengths (smaller frequencies), which correspond to the grave tones.

Because of this is that acoustic basses are large instruments, with a large body. Here, long-wavelength (and lower frequency) standing waves are generated. Violins otherwise have a small body, such that they can generate standing waves with short wavelengths (higher frequencies).

Actually, what happens in any musical instrument is that, when playing, not only one mode of oscillation is produced, but several of them are produced simultaneously. This is what gives that characteristic sound when of the execution of a note or a group of them (chord) in a particular instrument.

It is the so-called timbre of the instrument, which yields a special effect with a richness of sonorities when performing a group of instruments playing together, and which allows us to distinguish the origin of the sound produced by each one of them. Each instrument thus has its sonorous amplitude, corresponding to that frequency range in which it can generate a pattern of standing waves.

The wind musical instruments arose when the primitive men discovered that they could produce sounds when blowing some objects, like animal bones and bamboo. In general, they are formed by a tube, where the sound is produced by the passage of air in its interior. The larger and wider the tube, the more grave the sound it produces. The wind instruments are quite ancient and have been found in almost all primitive cultures. The flute is at least 40000 years old, and it has been found in virtually every culture on every continent.

When blowing a jet of air into the nozzle of a flute, the pressure inside the mouth is above atmospheric pressure. The air in the tube thus begins to vibrate, and some of the energy is radiated as sound, out of the open end as well as through the side holes. A significant amount of energy, however, is lost in the form of friction with the walls. When the note is sustained, this lost energy is replaced by the energy added by the performer.

The air column in the flute vibrates much more easily in some frequencies than in others, that is, it resonates at certain frequencies. These are determined by the length of the oscillating air column, and so the flutist can choose the desired effect by establishing the desired set of resonant frequencies by selecting a suitable combination of keys.

The flute is like a tube open at both ends. When observing someone playing, you will see that, although the person's lower lip covers part of the nozzle, part of the hole is open to the atmosphere. The open end means that the pressure is the atmospheric pressure, and then the acoustic pressure, i.e., the pressure variation due to the sound waves, is locally zero.

The air molecules are then free to enter and leave the open ends. These points are called pressure antinodes, and extend beyond the end of the tube by a small distance, about 0.6 times the radius of the cross-section. Inside the tube, the pressure is not atmospheric, and at the first resonance, the maximum pressure variation (antinode) occurs in the middle. The air jet has its natural frequency, which depends on its speed and length.

The flute usually develops a stronger resonance in the hole that is close to the natural frequency of the air jet. By putting a hole in the tube of a flute distant from one end, we construct a pressure antinode, which is equivalent to making the tube shorter. How the air flows into and out of the flute depends on the acoustic impedance of the nozzle. If the impedance is low, the air flows in and out immediately, and a loud sound can then be produced.

The resonances which are frequencies in which the acoustic impedance is small are very important, as they can better capture the behavior of the air jet, and so the flute will sound strongly at a frequency of resonance.

Most wind instruments have holes or keys that, when they are covered or tightened by the player's fingers, it is modified the space through which the air passes producing therein different musical notes. This category includes all the wind musical instruments whose sound is produced by the direct vibration of the performer's lips on a nozzle, as in the flutes, or on a single or double pallet, as in clarinet and oboe. The modern saxophone is also included in this family, an instrument built-in metal since its invention, but with a wooden pallet. All of them are made of metal alloys and have a very powerful sonority.

Other important representatives of this group are the horn, the trumpet, the trombone, and the tuba. All these are part of an orchestra as well as of military bands. The oldest instruments of this group had a smooth tube. Over time, additional holes, keys, and tubes have been added with threads and pistons.

The timpani are a percussion instrument based on the functioning of a vibrating membrane. This has a round head stretched over a closed box. The change in the membrane tension modifies the height of the emitted note. Its base is rounded and membrane can be adjusted with keys. The surface tension of the skin can be altered employing a pedal, which drives the tensioning clamping elements of the head.

The timpani membrane has a large number of modes of vibration. The fundamental mode is not the preferred one, because it is a muffled and not very pleasant sound. The percussionist musician chooses a point where he can emphasize the preferred modes of vibration of the circular membrane. The resulting frequencies are also influenced by the air-filled cavity.

The timpani were used by ancient civilizations in Asia, in the Mediterranean, in the African tribes and by the Indians of the Americas. It was introduced to Europe in the early 6th century, and being an instrument of great sonorous volume, was widely used in military bands and instrumental groups playing in open ambiances.

The earliest record of the use of timpani in Brazil dates back to the 18th century, in 1786, in the parade held in the center of Rio de Janeiro when of the celebration of the marriage of the Infantes D. João VI and D. Carlota Joaquina. In the 19th century, the timpani were already part of the music orchestras. After, in 1811, Father José Maurício Nunes Garcia composed a Hymn of Thanksgiving, in major C, for choir and orchestra, and in 1814 it was dedicated by the composer himself to the anniversary of the arrival of the Portuguese court in the city. In this, the use of the timpani is well valued.

The sound produced by the timpani is not generated by vibrations of a column of air or a string, but rather by a circular vibrating membrane. This does not vibrate in a harmonic series, i.e., the frequency of the higher modes are not integer multiples of the fundamental mode. Besides, since it vibrates in two dimensions, the timpani have two sets of nodal points: circles and lines (diameters). The nodal lines are formed by points that remain at rest, while the other parts of the membrane are vibrating. Unlike a string or a column of air, which vibrates in a single dimension, membranes vibrate in two dimensions.

The theory that describes how membranes vibrate has long been of interest to the scientific community. In the second half of the 18th century the Swiss mathematician and physicist Leonhard Euler (1707-1783) presented a treatise *De Motu Vibratorio Tympanorum* (On the movement of vibrations on drums) to the Berlin Academy, on January 22, 1761, and to the Petersburg Academy, May 17, 1762.

Subsequently, it was published in *Novi Commentarii Academiae Scientiarum Petropolitanae,* in 1766. This is the first known treatise dedicated to the science of a vibratory membrane.

Later, in the 18th century, the Italian scientist Giordano Ricatti (1709-1790) published his treatise *Delle vibrationi del tambour in Saggi scientifici and letterari dell'Academia di Padova,* in 1786.

Another important contribution came from the German physicist and musician Ernst Florens Friedrich Chladni (1756-1827), who invented a technique to show the various modes of vibration on a surface, the so-called patterns of Chladni, published in 1787 in his book *Entdeckungen uber die Theorie des Klanges* (Discoveries in Sound Theory).

In the mid-19th century, the German scientist and physicist Herman von Helmholtz derived an equation for the study of physical problems involving space and time and basic forms. The Helmholtz equation was applied to the circular membrane by the German mathematician Alfred Clebsch (1833-1872) in 1862. These works are the precursors to our current understanding of the mathematical functions of a vibrating membrane.

In a vibrating circular membrane the nodal lines, which are the points of minimum amplitude, are formed by straight lines (diameters) and circumferences. The first nodal region, found in mode (0,1), is located on an outer circumference, away from the center.

The nomenclature for the labeling of the modes is (d, c), where d is the number of nodal diameters (lines) and c is the number of nodal circumferences. For example, the second mode of vibration of a circular membrane is indicated as (1,1), which means that there is a diametral mode (the line running through the circle) and a circular mode. This is responsible for the characteristic tone of the timpani, and is called the main mode, but this is not the fundamental one.

The mode (0,1) of a drum, for example, is produced when it is struck at the center. When vibrating in this mode the membrane acts as a source that radiates the sound very effectively. However, the membrane quickly transfers its vibrational energy to the generated sound wave, so that the vibration ends quickly. The short duration (fraction of a second) of the mode $(0,1)$ means that it does not contribute much to the tone quality. In fact, upon being struck in the center, timpani (and other drums) produce a thud that decomposes rapidly.

Musical instruments are therefore devices we have created and adopted to control the oscillation of air in order to produce a vibratory pattern that greatly enriches the way of expressing our inner self, in a special language that affects and modifies the ambience in which we are, in order to create an atmosphere conducive to our well-being as well as of those around us.

3. Musical Scale

Archaeological studies of ancient civilizations bring evidence that the pursuit of understanding about different mechanisms for pleasantly producing sounds is a long-standing concern, which has also had much interest and support from the ruling classes.

Research on instrument design was already being developed in China and India in about 2000 BC, as indicated by records showing the study of musical scales. Also, the Arabs in antiquity studied subdivisions of the octave interval in the construction of a musical scale. It was in ancient Greece, however, that the concepts adopted in the Western world were created.

A musical scale is a group of notes arranged in sequence, from the lowest pitch to the highest one. This implies a fixed set of intervals within an octave. For example C D E F G A B C. The last C-note is one octave above the first and has a frequency equal to twice of it.

The earliest record shows the analysis of a musical scale dates from the 5th century BC in ancient Greece from the studies of Pythagoras (570-497 BC) on the mathematical relations between different tones. Before settling in southern Italy, Pythagoras traveled through Egypt and Babylon, where he probably had access to ancient knowledge about numbers. It is said that Pythagoras was a mystical person and that he could hear celestial music. Legend has it that he would have been inspired when hearing a blacksmith's hammer.

In his studies on sound intervals, Pythagoras experimented with a tensioned string (monochord) attached to the ends, mounted on adjustable support, with which he could control the length of the stretch on each side, and thus compare the sound effect produced by different lengths.

By placing the bracket halfway, he produced an octave, that is, a ratio of 2:1 in the frequency heard. By using different lengths and fingering along the two sides he could compare the effect of the consonance and the intervals of lengths in which the combination heard sounded pleasing to the ears. He thus constructed the so-called harmonic series and the consonant intervals. It is said that Pythagoras considered that such harmonic relations ruled the whole universe, and even spoke about *the Music of the Spheres*, referring to the celestial bodies. According to him, *everything vibrates*.

The specific frequencies used to construct a musical scale are not random. Some notes or intonations sound particularly well when played simultaneously.

Consonance is the combination of sound frequencies that sound pleasing to our hearing.

For an oscillating string attached at the ends, the vibratory pattern is that of transverse standing waves, that is, perpendicular vibrations in which the waveform does not move along the string. Thus, each point has well-defined amplitude. The positions of maxima (antinodes) and minimum (nodes) of the transverse displacements do not vary with time. At the ends, the transverse displacement is null (amplitude zero), which characterizes a node, whereas in the central part the fundamental mode of vibration has maximum transverse displacement, that is, an antinode.

Pythagoras initially noted that there was a pleasant combination of sounds when two stretched strings attached to the ends were percussed in such a way that the ratio of their lengths was 2:1 (octave interval) or 3:2 (perfect fifth). Given a fixed length, the speed of the wave depends also on the tension applied.

By varying the tension, the frequencies of the harmonic modes change. This is what happens when we tune the string of a guitar, for example. The harmonic series of vibrations on a string attached to the ends is given by $L = n\lambda/2$, where $n = 1,2,3...$ Hence, for a given L, the vibration frequencies of the harmonic modes are given by $f = nv/2L$. For each length, we have a frequency, for a given n value.

But these are inversely proportional quantities, i.e., when doubling one, the other is halved. Thus, by doubling the length of the string, the new frequency of vibration will be half of the previous one, that is, an octave below. On the other hand, if we divide the string in half, we will have a frequency equal to twice the initial frequency, i.e., an octave above. Musical notes that differ from each other by a factor of two have the same name. In the guitar, for example, when sounding the fourth loose string, we have the D note. If we press this string in the twelfth house, we still have the same note D but one octave above, i.e., with twice the frequency.

The Pythagorean scale is any scale constructed from the 3:2 and 2:1 frequency ratios, which correspond to the perfect fifth and octave intervals, respectively. Starting from note D, by multiplying its frequency by 3:2 gives the note A above it. If we proceed doing so, the next note above obtained by applying the factor 3:2 gives us the note E. However, this procedure does not allow a group of 3:2 intervals to fit exactly within one octave.

The Pythagorean scale based on the C note is obtained today exactly by the following frequency ratios: C (1) D (9/8) E (81/64) F (4/3) G (3/2) A(27/16) B (243/128) C (2). For a single string (monochord) the note G, which has a frequency at a ratio of 3/2 relative to the first note C at the beginning of the scale, corresponds to a length of 2/3 relative to it. For note F, this ratio is 4/3, which, for the same string, corresponds to a length of 3/4 of that one of the initial C note.

In ancient Greece, another musical scale was proposed by the astronomer Ptolemy, who added, to the relations 3:2:1 of Pythagoras, the 4:5:6 relations, where he observed that new consonances are obtained. For a scale starting with the C note, this results in the set of 4/4, 5/4, 6/4 = 1, 5/4, 3/2 intervals corresponding to the notes C, E, and G.

Or, equivalently, if the sound of a vibrating string of length L (4/4) is combined with those of two strings of 4/5 L and 4/6 L lengths, the combination sounds well to our ears. It turns out that this corresponds exactly to the so-called perfect chord (harmonic triad), formed by the third and fifth intervals, and added to the fundamental mode of vibration.

The chord C+ is thus formed by the three notes C, E, and G, corresponding to the tonic, supertonic and dominant notes of the diatonic scale of major C. In this scale, concerning the fundamental mode frequency C, the other frequency ratios are 9/8 (D), 5/4 (E), 4/3 (F), 3/2 (G), 5/3 (A) and 15/8 (B). The ratios 5/3 (= 20/12) and 15/8, corresponding to the highest frequencies, arising from the products of the ratios 5/4 and 4/3 by 3/2, respectively. It is interesting to note that in this way the largest interval between consecutive tones in this scale is the same as that of the Pythagorean scale (9/8), corresponding to one tone, while the shortest interval is slightly different (6.7%) from that of the Pythagorean scale (5.3%), although both are equivalent to a semitone.

These ancient scales are now known as fair intonation, equally tempered or of equal temperament.[7] However, when transposing a melody from one tonality to another, the need arises to introduce intermediate intervals, which do not exist in the Greek scales. This is done through the use of the accidents: sharp (#) and flat (♭) that raise or lower a note by 1/2 tone, respectively. In the Western system, on a 7-note scale, for example, from C to Si, including all the sharps, we have 12 consecutive semitones: C C# D D# E F F# G G# A A# B C.

Coma is also the designation of a musical interval, with the 1-tone interval comprising 9 commas, and then 1/2 tone corresponds to the range of 4.5 commas. Such intervals are only possible to be performed on instruments that have no frets, such as the violin, viola, and cello.

As notes that differ by a factor of 2 have the same name and considering that the natural range of an octave is divided into 12 strictly equal parts (semitones) in the temperate scale, this corresponds to the twelfth root of 2,

---

[7] Ross W. Duffin. How Equal Temperament Ruined Harmony (and Why You Should Care). W. W. Norton Company, Oct 2008.

that is, to $2^{1/12}$. Thus, for example, the note C (261.63 Hz) corresponds to $(2^{1/12})^0$. The note C# (277.18 Hz) is within the range of 4.5 commas above it, i.e., $(2^{1/12})^1 = 1.05946$, for the frequency ratio. The next note, D (293.67 Hz), is also 4.5 commas above the latter, i.e., in $(2^{1/12})^2 = 1.12246$, for the frequency ratio.

The first octave, which corresponds to twice the original frequency, is then (twelve semitones above) equal to $(2^{1/12})^{12} = 2$ (2:1 ratio). This is the tempered scale, which by its precise regularity, serves as the basis for comparing intervals with different scales in cases where there are even smaller units than a semitone, the so-called microtonal systems.

In the 16th century an Italian composer, Nicola Vicentino, constructed a keyboard that used 36 keys for an octave, to experiment micro intervals. In the last decades, the use of microtonal intervals has already been explored by several instrumentalists.

Thus, the frequency ratio between two consecutive notes is about 1.059 between semitones, and 1.122 per tone. With this, the C# equals the D ♭, the E# equals the F, and the F ♭ equals the E. Mathematically, an octave can also be divided into 1200 hundredths, such that if two tones differ by one hundredth, the ratio between their frequencies is $2^{1/1200} = 1.0005777$. The distinguishing threshold of the human hearing is approximately 2 cents.

Any interval smaller than this is not perceived by most people.

Each musical scale has its characteristic sonority. In the tempered system, the musical intervals are the same, and this is commonly used for instrument tuning. One of the advantages of this scale is that it remains unchanged throughout the whole musical range so that compositions can be freely transposed up or down without changing intervals.

Currently, the equal temperament scale is the standard in Western music. The piano keyboard is the classical example of the equal temperament scale. The natural notes (C D E F G A B) are represented on the piano by the white keys, while the black keys represent the intermediate notes (semitones). The frets of a modern guitar are also arranged to create on the instrument the equal temperament scale.

In the chromatic scale, an octave has 12 semitones, and two notes distant by a semitone, such as C and C# constitute a minor second interval, whereas an interval of two semitones forms a major second. Other intervals are the minor third, third, perfect fourth, tritone, perfect fifth, minor sixth, major sixth, minor seventh, major seventh and octave. Therefore, all scales are thus subsets of the chromatic scale. Some scales may have 5, 6 or 8 notes, but most of them have 7 notes.

A chord is a set of notes played simultaneously. The simplest chord is a harmonic triad, that is, composed of three notes separated by one-third intervals. From C to E we have a major third, and from E to G, a minor third. On a 7-note scale, we have the sequence: tonic, supertonic, subdominant, dominant, super dominant, sensitive, and octave.

The semitones are classified as chromatic or diatonic. Between two adjacent notes, as E-F, this is diatonic and corresponds to a minor second interval. A chromatic semitone is the one in which the notes have the same names, like C and C #.

The difference between the chromatic and diatonic semitones is a single coma, which is practically impossible for the human ear to distinguish. The chromatic semitone has 4 commas and the diatonic 5 commas. In the system of the equal temperament scale, the semitones are considered equal, with 4,5 commas.

In the diatonic scale of major C, some intervals are equal to 9/8 of the scale, such as C-D, F-G, and A-B, whereas the D-E and G-A intervals are slightly smaller (10/9), which differ by a comma. The E-F and B-C intervals are slightly bigger than a semitone, but with a difference smaller than one coma, and equal to 16/15. The notes changed by the accidents sharp (#) and flat (♭) are formed from the multiplication or division of the original note by 25/24, respectively. So the seven-note scale becomes one of the twenty-one notes if we include two accidents per note, i.e., C ♭ , C and C#.

In the mid-19th century, with the evolution of the piano, the equal temperament scale spread out and became worldwide adopted. However, musicians and lovers of the "good temperament" did not like the isochromatic properties of the equal temperament. Although this latter is widely used today in the Western world, in an orchestra there are still instruments that are precise by nature and do not use the equal temperament, and thus is rather preferred to play the flats than the sharps. Among these are the instruments of the family of violins, violas, cellos, trombones and even the human voice.

When composing a song one usually chooses a scale, and a general trend is to use the notes of this scale. A note played out of this range sounds as out of key. Each musical note has its own set of scales, for example, major, minor, pentatonic, etc. The scales of major and minor tones are differentiated by the sequence of tones and semitones that composes them.

In the major C diatonic scale, for example, the sequence of tones and semitones is 2 tones 1 semitone 3 tones 1 semitone. All major diatonic scales have this same sequence of tones and semitones. There are several types of scale, some of which are more suitable for different musical styles, such as jazz, blues, old, baroque and medieval music. Jazz improvisation is based on harmonic progressions, that is, on a sequence of chords.

The musical scale is the most explicit representation of the harmonic view of the mathematics of numbers, where numerical reasons represent vibrational modes that translate into pleasant sonorous sensations in our ears, whose combinations permeate our innermost feelings and lead our sensations into modulations of a higher spiritual state.

4. Hearing

When we listen to music, the sound waves that cause the vibrations in the air reach our ear generating physical reactions that are translated into nerve impulses and electrical signals. These communicate to the brain a bunch of information that we are still far from fully understanding. But in our mind are recorded a variety of patterns corresponding to the different types of sound we hear.

All this information remains integrated into our body using complex mechanisms, and as a consequence, all functions in our organism can be affected in some way through the nervous system. A young, healthy human being can hear sounds in the range 20-2000 Hz with a resolution of about 0.2% in frequency, which means distinguishing the difference between sounds of 1000 and 1002 Hz.

Sounds below 20 Hz are classified as subsonic, and those above 2000 0 Hz are called ultrasounds. Older people or people with conviviality with high sonorous levels usually lose their hearing for higher frequencies. On the other hand, the good news is that most of a normal conversation is below 2000 Hz.

The average frequency range of the human voice is between 120 and 1100 Hz. The strident crying of a newborn is between about 2000 and 3000 Hz, which is close to the frequency of greater sensitivity of the human hearing, not by chance.

The vowels are grouped around frequencies between 300 and 750 Hz. Some consonants have very low frequencies, less than 250 Hz, while others can have frequencies as high as 3000 and 8000 Hz, produced speechless and in a whistling way, by blowing air between the teeth.

The human ear is incredibly sensitive. The threshold of our hearing corresponds to a sound wave intensity of 10^{-12} Watts/m^2. The human hearing does not follow a linear scale, that is, if the sound intensity doubles, it is not twice as loud. To be twice as loud, the sound intensity must be ten times higher!

In the field of acoustics, we also study how to extract important information about the propagation of sound in the ambiance, whether form voice or musical communication, as well as in defense situations, when there is some kind of threat or danger.

Strident sound effects were used by primitive men to frighten animals, and in the ancient battlefields yells of wind instruments and loud noises were used to elevate the morale of the troops and to intimidate the enemy. In the primitive tribes, the evolution of musical instruments began when one noticed that tensioned strings produced interesting and pleasant sounds when percussed, as well as the sound of strokes on animal skins, stretched and dried out.

The understanding of the mechanism of functioning of the human hearing has always aroused everyone's curiosity and is still a subject of deep study to physiologists, and the findings continue to evolve. The hearing mechanism is a rather complex system with several subdivisions.

The processing by the brain of the auditory stimuli is still too intricate and poorly understood. An acknowledged pioneering and highly relevant work was done by Georg von Békésy (1899-1972) who received the Nobel Prize in Medicine for his discoveries on the physical stimulus mechanism and the selectivity of frequencies in the inner ear.

Upon hearing a 1 kHz sound the eardrum shifts from about 1 Å (angstrom, or 10^{-10} m), which is roughly the diameter of a hydrogen atom. The ear picks up the sound from the outside like a microphone retransmitting signals through the nervous system to the brain. The ear is subdivided into three main areas: the outer, middle and inner regions. The outer ear is the external portion responsible for capturing the sound and transmitting it through a canal to the middle ear.

The middle ear is the part where sound waves are transformed into mechanical vibrations to be transmitted to the next part, the inner ear, where vibrations stimulate receptors, which in turn convert them into nerve impulses that go to the central nervous system by the acoustic nerve.

The outer ear comprises the auricle (or ear), the external acoustic meatus and the tympanic membrane. The main function of the auditory canal is the collection of sounds, which are directed to the ear canal. The external acoustic meatus connects the pavilion to the eardrum, which is a flat channel, with rigid walls, constantly open. The outermost part of this canal has elastic cartilage, which is the continuation of the cartilage of the auricular pavilion[8].

The acoustic meatus is lined with hairs, sebaceous and ceruminous glands. The secretion of these glands is called cerumen, a darkened pasty substance, which has a protective function to hinder the entry of foreign bodies, as well as to prevent against moisture that facilitates the installation of bacteria in the ear that causes infection.[9].

[8]L.C. Junqueira. Histologia Básica: Texto y Atlas. 2015.
[9], Pierre Buser. Audition (Bradford Books) The MIT Press, Jun. 1992.

At the bottom of the meatus is the eardrum, an oval-shaped membrane, covered by a thin skin. The auditory canal has the function of transmitting the sounds captured by the ear to the tympanic membrane, acting as a resonance chamber to amplify the signal. This membrane transmits the vibrations to the ossicles (smaller bones of the human body) of the middle ear.

The middle ear is a space of the temporal bone filled by air, located between the eardrum and the inner ear, formed by the ossicles hammer, anvil, stirrup and auditory tube, also called Eustachian tube, which communicates with the pharynx.

Usually, the auditory tube is closed, but it opens during chewing, swallowing and yawning so that the external pressure is balanced with the middle ear. The sensation of pressure in the ears is perceived during the flights or in situations of changes of altitude, caused by this process of balancing pressure.

Mammals are the only animals that have three bones in the ear, connecting the eardrum to the inner ear. The main function of the middle ear is to transmit the vibrations of the tympanum to the fluid-filled structures of the inner ear.

The sound waves make vibrate the tympanic membrane, which in turn moves the ossicles through a system of levers that produce mechanical vibrations to be detected and converted into nerve impulses. The auditory tube helps to maintain the balance of air pressure between the tympanic cavity and the external surroundings.

The inner ear is called labyrinth and is a complex structure made up of membranes filled with fluid, housed within cavities in the hardened part of the temporal bone. The bony labyrinth is formed by a central cavity of irregular shape, the vestibule, which is in the posterior part and is related to the balance, and the cochlea or snail, in the anterior part, related to the hearing.

The last bone of the ossicular chain is the stapes, which is attached to a thin membrane (oval window) which is an entrance to the inner ear, which contains the organ of hearing. When the stirrup moves, the oval window moves along with it. On the other side of the oval window is the cochlea, a snail-shaped channel, filled with a liquid, which is agitated by the movements of the oval window.

When the vibrations reach the cochlea these are transformed into compression waves, which in turn activate the organ of Corti, formed by thousands of ciliated cells that move every time the liquid is shaken.

The acoustic energy of sound waves leads to the stimulation of these cells, which generates electrical impulses that are then sent to the brain. Some problems with the semicircular canals can result in symptoms such as vertigo. The diffraction of sound waves inside the head affects balance and the sensation of comfort or discomfort.

Sound waves are directed by the auricle pavilion to the ear canal. Any changes in air pressure due to the passage of a sound wave reach the tympanum, which begins to vibrate. As the hammer cable is attached to it, the ossicles' structure is vibrated. This system acts as a transformer, modifying the energy collected by the tympanum.

The sound stimulus picked up by the ear then enters the ear canal, which is a tube about 0.75 cm in diameter and 2.5 cm in length. This channel terminates in the tympanic membrane. Under the impulse of sound waves, this begins to vibrate and transmitting the vibrations through a system of small bones connected to the ossicular chain: the hammer, the anvil, and the stirrup.

It is estimated that almost a quarter of the world population between the ages of 15 and 75 suffers from hearing loss. This can be caused by infectious diseases or excessive exposure to loud noises, or then simply, come with aging. Most people, as they get older, lose hearing at higher frequencies, and this progressively goes downwards. Thus, the sounds of the consonants are the first to be lost, and these are the ones that usually distinguish similar sounds. Vowels have a higher sound level.

This is why many senior people say they listen to people talking but cannot understand what they are saying. The main problem with hearing loss is the difficulty of discerning well a conversation and a person's ability to understand speech. It can even happen that a child's school performance is adversely affected by hearing difficulties.

For a sound to be audible the amplitude of the waves must be above the hearing threshold, which defines the transition between audibility and inaudibility. When the amplitude of the sound exceeds this limit, it is processed and perceived as having certain qualities like volume, tone, and timbre. The study of the auditory perception concerning the physical characteristics of sound comprises the field of psychoacoustics.

The wide range of frequencies of the sound waves present in nature creates an acoustic ambiance unknown to us. Our ear is not equally sensitive to all frequencies. This depends on a variety of factors, the most important being the level of sound pressure and frequency. A sound of 30 Hz and a sound level of 95 dB can be judged by a listener to be as equally loud as a sound of 1000 Hz and 70 dB, or even as a sound of 5000 Hz and 65 dB.

However, the higher the sound level, the greater the physiological discomfort, which can range from a simple itch to the sensation of pain. The pain threshold is at 120 dB, but different people have different tolerances for high volume noise, and therefore have different thresholds for painful sensation, although these do not differ much from the statistical averages for healthy young ears.

The adult male voice has on average a fundamental frequency between 120 and 150 Hz, while the adult female voice typically lies between 210 and 240 Hz. In general, animals can hear sounds in a wider range of frequencies comparatively to humans. While our average hearing is in the range of 20-20000 Hz, whales can perceive sounds in the range of approximately 0.5-125000 Hz, with a sensitivity peak around 20000 Hz. Bats' hearing sweeps an interval of 10-100000 Hz.

Elephants have exceptional senses of smell and hearing. They can hear frequencies twenty times lower than us. They also use their trunk and feet to listen, both of which are equipped with special receivers to pick up low-frequency vibrations. Their hearing ability allows them to perceive approaching storms and explains the well-known fact that elephants are always the first animals to move in case of rain, earthquakes, and tsunamis. Their screams can be heard by other elephants 6 km away.

An elephant is very sensitive to low-frequency sounds too and can hear a 16-Hz sound at a level of 65 dB. However, the elephant is insensitive to sounds above 12000 Hz. There appears to be an inverse correlation between head size and auditory acuity for high frequencies in terrestrial mammals. Psychophysical investigations in birds indicate for these a region of maximum sensitivity between 1 and 5000 Hz.

The owl has a phenomenal hearing. Their large ear holes are at slightly different heights, above and below eye level, helping them to identify the vertical positions of the sound sources. But what is truly amazing is their reaction time. In complete darkness, an owl takes about less than 0.01 seconds to assess the precise direction of a running mouse.

Bats and dolphins can find their way in complete darkness. Bats can detect the presence of a flying insect 20 meters away. Dolphins can navigate in murky waters using a biological sonar system, emitting ultrasonic whistles and interpreting echoes of sound waves received back. They can spot a coin 70 meters away.

Pigeons can hear sounds of extremely low frequencies and this helps to explain their exceptional sense of direction. Steep slopes can reflect sound waves horizontally thus allowing pigeons to orient themselves over large distances. The pigeons also have the equivalent of an internal compass, which allows them to navigate using the Earth's magnetic field and the position of the sun. All this, combined with their hearing, makes them the best navigators in nature.

Not only can cats listen to higher frequencies than dogs and humans, but they can still distinguish the tone as well as locate its source even much better. With 30 different muscles, the cat can independently rotate each ear by 180-degrees, and the position of one ear or both, and besides, thanks to its shape, the sound is channeled to the middle ear much more effectively.

The auditory property of our ears enriches formidably our perception of the outside world and conducts directly into our brain and nervous system the sensations of what happens around us far beyond we can see, which permeates into our body and soul the vibrations of the sonorous ambiance.

5. Acoustics

Since ancient times it must have been perceived the influence of the surroundings in the way we hear a speech addressed to an audience. The project of the Roman amphitheaters shows that there was already knowledge of the need to adapt the building to improve the hearing of the spectacles.

This is the field of studies of the acoustics, which deals with the production and transmission of sound through different materials, the reverberation in closed ambient as well as the effects of sound waves on living beings.

From a purely mechanical effect, the sound is essentially the incidence of pressure fluctuations resulting from the oscillatory forces acting on the constituent particles of a medium. Sound plays a major role in our lives, and for this reason, the science of acoustics is very old.[10]

The precursor of the modern megaphone was used by Alexander the Great of Macedonia (400 BC) to summon

---

[10] Richard E Berg and David G Stork. The Physics of Sound, 3rd Edition. Pearson, 2004.

his troops on the battlefields. The Roman engineer-architect Vitruvius in 25 BC proposed a model based on the propagation of circular waves on the surface of the water to explain how sound should propagate in the air, not as circles but as spherical waves. He was also known for using a linear distribution of empty bronze vases to improve the acoustics of large rooms. These would have the effect of absorbing low-frequency sounds in a way similar to that of special panels today used as sound absorbers for better acoustics of ambiances.

The direct propagation of sound and its reflection on surfaces were also studied by the ancient civilizations. Studies on acoustics were carried out by the Greek philosopher Chrysippus in about 240 BC, and by the Roman philosopher Severino Boethius (480-524 AD). The great Greek philosopher Aristotle (384-322 BC) noted that the movement of the air which occurs with the passage of sound causes a push forward onto a surface.

Also in Greece Pythagoras (570-497 BC) observed that the movement of air generated by a vibrating object produces a musical note with the same frequency of the vibrating body. Pythagoras then sought to apply mathematics to describe intervals and musical consonances.

Already at the Renaissance, Leonardo da Vinci (1452-1519) noted the need for a medium for the propagation of sound. He also tried to correlate the waves generated on the surface of the water with the sound propagation, considering that this latter could be a similar wave phenomenon. He argued that the movement of sound waves happens at a well-defined speed.

Da Vinci further noted that the ringing of a bell is answered by a small vibration from another bell in the vicinity, just as the sound of the vibrating strings of a lute vibrated the instrument as a whole at the same frequency, causing similar vibrations in another lute nearby.

The property of sound in circling obstacles also was known in antiquity. Whispering galleries, which come from a sound effect of the wind in cavities and openings, were used as a distraction in the medieval castles and palaces.

In the ancient texts, there are records of bizarre procedures, such as recommending music as a treatment for spider bites, as well as studies on the effect of sound on both young and aged wines, and even on the possibility of imprisoning the sound in a box.

However, no significant progress in acoustics was recorded until the 17th century, when a relationship between a sonorous field and frequency was finally established by the French philosopher and Franciscan Friar Marin Mersenne (1588-1648), considered the father of modern acoustics. Mersenne even measured the speed of sound by counting the number of heartbeats during the interval between the flash of a gunshot and the perception of the sound bang.

The Italian Galileo Galilei (1564-1642), independently, in his work *Discorsi su due nuove scienze*, published in 1638, already discussed notions of frequency. An alternative concept to that of waves for sound was conceived by Pierre Gassendi (1582-1655), a contemporary of Galileo and Mersenne, who defended the theory that sound is attributed to a stream of atoms emitted by the vibrating body. The velocity of sound would then be the speed of moving particles, and frequency would be the number of particles emitted per unit time.

In 1660 in England Robert Boyle (1626-1691) performed experiments that indeed confirmed the need for air to propagate sound. The German physicist and musician Ernst Florenz Friedrich Chladni (1756-1827), investigated vibrations in membranes and calculated the sound velocity in different gases using stems and resonant tubes. In the 17th century, with the advancement of knowledge about wave phenomena, the concepts of refraction, diffraction, and interference were also applied to sound.

Diffraction is the scattering of a wave that occurs when it meets an obstacle with dimensions comparable to its wavelength. When two waves meet, there can be two types of patterns of interference, constructive and destructive. Constructive interference occurs when two waves are added such as to reinforce the vibrating signal. Destructive interference occurs when two incoming waves are completely out of phase and cancel each other.

In the 19th century, the English mathematician and physicist John William Strutt (1842-1919), also known as Lord Rayleigh, developed important studies in wave phenomena that yielded the theoretical foundations of modern acoustics.

Until the early 12th century the ships were warned of dangerous conditions utilizing floating bells. The development of ultrasound came from the need for ships to avoid dangerous submerged obstacles. In 1916 it was already possible to obtain echoes of the bottom of the ocean until a distance of about 200 m. Later on, the first devices were produced to generate directional beams of acoustic energy with the use of ultrasound.

In architecture, the study of acoustics allowed the development of more appropriate materials to adapt the walls of a room to improve the ambient acoustics.[11] In the United States, Harvey Fletcher (1884-1981), considered the father of psychoacoustics, led research to describe and

---

[11]Daniel R. Raichel. The Science and Applications of Acoustics (Aip Series in Modern Acoustics and Signal Processing.). Springer, 2000.

quantify the concepts of volume and the determinant factors for voice communication. Fletcher developed the first electronic hearing aid equipment at Bell Laboratories and was the creator of the stereo reproduction.

More and more advanced technologies are being developed to produce images of vibrations of the body of musical instruments and machines, as well as to investigate the propagation of sound waves at very low (cryogenic) temperatures and to analyze the vibrational modes of elastic bodies.

Ultrasound devices today are used to obtain fetal imaging, to dislodge dental plaques, to overcome the effects of atherosclerosis, to release clogged blood vessels, to provide non-invasive medical diagnoses, to aid in surgical procedures and to provide a means of nondestructive testing of materials. They are employed for cleaning almost everything using vibrations, from precious stones to clogged pipes. Nowadays current computerized noise-canceling techniques are used to neutralize excessive noise in aircraft, submarines, and automobiles.[12]

Reverberation consists of the persistence of a sound even after its emission from the source is extinguished. This occurs due to reflections on the walls and surfaces of a

---

[12]Harry F. Olson. Music, Physics, and Engineering (Dover Books on Music). Dover Publications, 1967.

room. In some closed ambient, undesirable reflections and excessive reverberations can very damagingly mask the sound of a speech. There is a relation between the quality of the acoustics, the dimensions of a chamber and the number of absorption surfaces present.

The reverberation time is defined as the number of seconds required for the sound intensity to drop from an audibility level of 60 dB, above the hearing threshold, to the verge of inaudibility. The reverberation time is still the most important parameter used to measure the acoustic quality of a room. This can be reduced by strategically spreading panels of materials with good absorption throughout the ambient.[13]

The placement of absorbent surfaces in an ambient allows a listener to perceive predominantly the sound emitted directly from the source, free from the multiple reflections on the walls. A free field then can be simulated in a given ambiance if all the surrounding surfaces are coated with absorbent materials, thus eliminating the presence of undesirable echoes.

The combination of various surfaces in an auditorium amplification system is used to achieve better diffusion. This can be achieved by placing special baffle

---

[13] Menezes, FLO. Acústica Musical em Palavras e Sons, A. Martins Fontes, 2014.

panels hanging from the ceiling to divert the sonorous waves along with appropriate directions. The panels should not be aligned or parallel, so there is no preferred direction for the sound propagation.

The sound that reaches a listener indirectly has less intensity than that which comes directly from the source because the reflected path is longer than the direct source-listener distance. This results in greater divergence and loss of intensity due to the absorption occurring in the surfaces along the way.

The indirect sound that a listener perceives comes from a larger number of reflection paths, which leads to the degeneration of the signal quality. If the walls of the room are good absorbers, there are no echoes, and the situation approaches that one of a free field. When the source suddenly ceases emission, a sound field can remain for a short time as a result of multiple reflections, and this, allied to the low propagation velocity of the sound, causes, in turn, a residual acoustic signal, called reverberant field.

The presence of reverberation tends to mask the immediate perception of direct sound. Short reverberation time is required to minimize echo effects so that a speech can be easily understood. A longer reverberation time otherwise contributes to making a weak signal more audible. On the other hand, an extremely short reverberation time tends to make the music sound harder, less musical, that is, less enjoyable. However, excessively long reverberation time makes it difficult to distinguish between different musical notes.

The adjustment of this parameter depends on the volume and extension of the room, and thus an adequate value represents an optimization between the two extremes. With the absorption in the walls and surfaces of a room, there is a reduction of the reverberation time. Harder surfaces such as ceramic tile floors and mirrors tend to prolong it. Also, walls should provide good insulation against external noise to improve the quality of the sound produced in an auditorium.

Absorption in the walls and surfaces of the ambient, however, prevents the sound intensity from becoming infinitely high. In an auditorium project, it is desirable that many audience members are as close as possible to the source, as sound levels tend to decrease with increasing distances from the emitter. A good visual line of the stage usually results in good acoustics.

The distribution of acoustic energy in a room, whether it comes from single or multiple sources, depends on the size and geometric shape of the ambient as well as on the combined effects of reflection, diffraction, and absorption. In the approximation of a punctual source, there is a free field in the region around it, wherein the sound pattern occurs as in an open space.

From the punctual source, the emitted wavefronts are spherical surfaces, and the intensity decreases with the propagation following the square inverse law. However, the presence of obstacles along the path of the waves, as well as the dimensions of the room, will interfere with their progression.

To eliminate exterior noises it can be used thick or even multiple walls. A ventilation system can also be quite noisy, and it needs to have adequate sound insulation, promoting a large displacement of air at low speed thereof minimizing undesirable noises and vibrations.

In domes and vaults, the diffusion of sound on curved surfaces also causes deformation of the sound waves and consequent alteration in the local acoustics. The presence of concave surfaces, with radii of curvature comparable to the wavelengths, tends to cause the focusing of the waves, while convex surfaces promote their diffusion.

A diffusion field can be established via a large number of reflected or diffracted waves that combine to uniformly distribute the sonorous energy in the room. Acoustic shells are economical structures for creating a more conducive ambiance for outdoor musical performances. However, soil topology is also crucial for achieving adequate acoustics.

In the exhibition of a symphonic orchestra in an auditorium the sound waves are reflected in the walls and objects of the room, and they will then spread out until the intensity of the sound reaches a level of balance, i.e., what is emitted minus what is absorbed reaches a situation of equilibrium, and the sound intensity remains constant therefrom.

For a lecture room, the project must take into account more places for listeners on the direct path of sound, so that the articulation clarity of successive syllables is sustained. Rooms for musical ambiances may have slightly longer reverberation times, but one still needs to avoid acoustic defects, such as echoes, particularly those from the back wall of the room. These can be diminished or even eliminated by the placement of panels with an appropriate arrangement, absorbing surfaces on the walls as well as irregularities in the surfaces to promote a good diffusion of the sound. In small rooms, the continuous reflection of sound waves between parallel and opposing walls can greatly impair the acoustic quality of the ambient.

Generally, three basic forms are followed in the design of large auditoriums: rectangular, tapered and horseshoe.[14] The rectangular hall is quite traditional and is

---

[14]Thomas D. Rossing and Neville H. Fletcher. Sound in concert halls and studios. In Principles of Vibration and Sound, pages 251–276. Springer New York, 2004.

suitable to accommodate both small and large audiences. But these rooms always generate cross-reflections and echoes between parallel walls. Sound can also be reflected off the back walls depending on their shape and degree of absorption. However, such reflections can sometimes provide a reasonable degree of diffusion in rooms of modest dimensions.

In a considerably larger room, resonances and standing wave modes with excessive vibration may occur, in addition to the presence of echoes. A project aimed at superior acoustics thus takes into account a relatively small size, high ceiling, and irregular plaster-lined interior surfaces. A fan-shaped room accommodates a larger audience, closer to the stage. It is often necessary to add a series of internal reflectors or panels hung on the ceiling over a certain area to maintain the acoustic characteristics.

The horseshoe shape has been widely used as the preferred design for modest opera houses and concert halls. This project provides a greater sense of intimacy and the convex surfaces promote proper sound diffusion. Multiple balconies also allow for an excellent line of sight, and a short distance for direct sound. The *La Scala* Opera House in Milan, opened in 1778, is probably the most notable example of the horseshoe project. Other examples are the Carnegie Hall in New York, completed in 1897, and the Academy of Music, the first opera house in the United States, inaugurated in 1857 in Philadelphia.

Particularly after World War II, there has been an accelerated development of research in acoustics, given the demand for new technologies, such as to enable voice communication in high noise surroundings such as aircraft cabins, in armored vehicles and industry. Today acoustics also plays an important role in medicine and chemistry, since some chemical reactions have been observed to occur upon accelerated reaction paths under certain acoustic conditions. Nowadays is observed an increasing number of studies on the physiological effects of sound in living organisms.

Acoustics represents the response of an object or environment to the presence of sound fields that introduce modes of vibration which propagate and reverberate throughout the ambiance, affecting incisively everything and everyone who witnesses the sound emission.

6. The Psyche of the Music

Throughout history, since ancient times, several musical movements have taken place and the records that have come to our knowledge help us to delineate the social structure characteristic of that era. It is the case of Medieval, Renaissance, Baroque, Classical, Romantic ages, and so on, and today, most of what we know best about the musical compositions of the past represents what the nobility and the religious elite enjoyed in social events. Of profane music, one knows almost nothing, as well as of that one appreciated in the ancient Roman and Egyptian civilization. Fortunately, some instruments survived the time and we can then have a vague idea of the musical sonority practiced in the past.

With the evolution of the media in the modern world, the dissemination of musical creations allowed an intense cultural exchange, where, even though scattered throughout the whole world, diverse groups of quite different social movements can enjoy and share similar tastes and musical preferences. These artistic manifestations are today well-delineated records of the social climate and behavior changes that accompany the twists of customs over time.

One who sings or plays an instrument can instantaneously transmit to the surroundings the feelings that he experiences at that precise moment. The sonority thus produced carries in its expression a theme with a significance imbued with varied emotions that can sensitize the hardest hearts, and which has the power to create an emotion-laden mood. This does not pass unnoticed by the living beings in the surroundings, and each one in its own way experiences some kind of commotion relatively to the perceived sound.

Music is an art language and a way of expression of the human unconscious, where the author seeks to imbue sounds with emotions and feelings. The listener experiences an altered state of consciousness of a profoundly particular meaning, defined by his sensitivity and identification with the original stimulus. The effect has an unpredictable outcome, but more and more discussion of its therapeutic character has been brought to the forefront of the scientific studies.

A melodic and pleasant musical trail easily can lead us to a state of melancholy and nostalgia or otherwise to euphoria and desire to dance. This depends on the rhythm, the emotional content of the song, the surroundings where we find ourselves, but it also depends very much on our mood at the moment, the situations we are experiencing in our daily lives as well as our ongoing affective relations.

Still, what pleases some, will not necessarily please everyone.

Music contributes to the process of manifestation of the inner self, as it serves as a way of expressing the voice of the unconscious, and thus represents a way that a person finds to say what does not commonly appear in his speech.[15] It has a property that transcends the intellect and that represents a manner for altering consciousness, which in turn can help us to some extent to practice self-control and reach emotional balance, which promotes physical health, bring happiness and is a prerequisite for personal well-being and growth.

The power that music has to deal with our emotions and feelings, gives it a certain therapeutic character, as an auxiliary resource in treatment procedures not only for the diseases of the physical body but also in cases of deviations of behavior and critical situations of emotional disturbances.

Psyche is a Greek word used to describe the soul or spirit. The unconscious and music can be related from the perspective of analytical psychology, as a stimulus to the transcendence of consciousness, favoring the evocation of

---

[15] Música Compõe O Homem E O Homem Compõe a Música, Gregório José Pereira De Queiroz Editora Cultrix.

images from the psyche, reducing in this manner the ego defenses.[16]

This form of expression, which uses a language not only verbal, can induce relaxation and help the passage to an altered state of consciousness that contributes definitely to enrich the therapeutic process.

In the 19th century, the French psychologist Gustave Le Bon (1841-1900) addressed in his studies the subjects of mass psychology, herd behavior and theories about national characteristics and race superiority. He proposed the concept of a psychological group, where the individuals develop a common characteristic, the so-called collective mind. This causes an individual to acquire distinct and incoherent mental and behavioral characteristics when compared to those that he would normally present if observed individually.

In his studies, the Austrian Sigmund Freud (1856-1939), neurologist and founder of psychoanalysis, points out that group psychology is interested in the individual as a member of a race, a nation, a caste, a profession, an institution, or as a part of a multitude of people who have organized themselves into a group on a

---

[16] Julio César Nunes Ito, Revista da Sociedade Brasileira de Psicologia Analitica, v. 36-1. p.9-18, 2018.

specific occasion for a definite purpose. [17] Freud emphasizes, however, that for a group to be formed, there must be a common ground that enables the coalition, i.e., something that represents a communion of interests and an emotional bond. In this context, it presents the theory of libido, an expression extracted from the theory of emotions.

This is the name given to instinctual psychic energy derived from primitive biological urges, considered as a quantitative but not measurable magnitude of those instincts that have to do with everything that can be covered under the word love. However, according to him, the core of what we mean by love naturally consists of sexual love, having sexual union as its goal.

An emotional bond, however, sometimes even of a sexual nature, can even be strengthened among people who share the same taste for a musical style, and the emotional bond thus strengthens, even more, worshiping the fashions and behavior of that person whose admiration and idolatry is a reference in society. A collective empathy around the object of the ego is then established through a process of identification, which contributes to the organization of the group, bringing together individuals with the most varied differences around a common point, with tribal characteristics.

---

[17] The Ego and the Id. Sigmund Freud. Courier Dover Publications, Mar 21. 2018 Psychology.

For Freud, the subject consists of a being whose personal and psychic characteristics are constructed and developed from his interaction with other subjects within different social groups. In the mode of the social interactions that each person develops throughout his life, several complex psychic mechanisms are created and assimilated, thus defining a very individual character profile for the feelings experienced by each one in his affective, family and social ties.

In this sense, music poses itself as an authentic way of dealing with the unconscious psychic processes that are produced through the interaction of the individual with the different social groups. In Freudian psychoanalysis, *the drive* is the psychic energy that directs action to an end, exhausting itself when achieving it. This is the psychic representative of an endosomatic (bodily) source of stimulation that flows continuously, unlike the stimulus, produced through excitations from external sources.

As an expression of the unconscious, music is thus a language that allows the individual to use metaphors and subjective and personalized linguistic symbols that reside in the depths of the author's unconscious.[18] This form of language allows the subject to express emotions, feelings,

---

[18] Fritz Winckel. Music, Sound, and Sensation: A Modern Exposition (Dover Books on Physics). Dover Publications, May 2012.

ideas and latent contents as a way of communicating with the world around us.

It is interesting to note that sentiments that are revived by recalling events that have a strong emotional content lead the author of a musical piece to compose a particular melody, and that, when appreciated by someone, evokes memories of special past moments loaded with sentimentalism, awakened by the same melody but with a completely different meaning.

Those who hear a beautiful melody perceive the awakening of a plurality of emotions that trigger a wide variety of sensations, sometimes of strong emotive meaning. It is indeed a language imbued with sentimentality created by the author, reinvented by the interpreter, and that in its transmission and communication, whether live or recorded, awakens in those who are listening to it a bunch of sensations, commotions and images capable of sparking quite different feelings far beyond those experienced by the composer, independently of time.

In the precise moment of the listening, according to the complexity of the daily routine experienced by each one, and the ambiance in which one lives, the triggering of emotions associated with memories introduces the most unexpected and differentiated consequences in every person, anytime and everywhere. Besides, changes in rhythm, the timbre of the voice or instrument, combined with different arrangements, introduce even more diverse effects in the listener, compared to the original composition.

According to the Swiss psychiatrist Carl Gustav Jung (1875-1961), founder of analytical psychology, the psyche is composed of three levels: conscious, personal unconscious and the collective unconscious. The interaction between conscious and unconscious determines the personality of a person.

In 1956, after a meeting with a pianist and music therapist, Jung acknowledges that music should be an important part of any analysis. He, who once used to view music therapy as sentimental and superficial, after experiencing a treatment with a pianist, recognized that the use of music for therapeutic purposes opened new routes of research in a perspective that he had never considered before.

The act of experiencing the therapy using musical sounds allowed him to contact deep contents of the psyche, thus opening up new possibilities in psychotherapy.[19] In his work The Nature of Psyche, Jung observes how an acoustic stimulus is capable of evoking images of the psyche, explaining that when an indefinite sound is heard,

---

[19] Carl Gustav Jung Editora Vozes Limitada, Mar 4, 2011. Psychology.

it summons a series of representations that unfold in acoustic, visual images and sensory. For him, the psyche is composed of images.

Music can then be understood as an objectification of the spirit, which favors the evocation of latent contents of the psyche not accessible to consciousness, and that can more easily pass through the blockages into the inner world of emotions and feelings. Music has thus unpredictable but positive effects on the body, psyche, and mind of the listener.

The beneficial effect of classical music on people, plants and animals are already recognized by many. Such an effect is powerful on our feelings and mood, and although incontrovertible, its mechanism remains practically unknown. Nevertheless, it is known that when listening to a pleasing musical trail a neurochemical alteration occurs accompanied by a discharge of dopamine. This is a powerful neurotransmitter that plays a key role in inducing and maintaining the body's necessary activities, such as food consumption and sex, and which is also known as responsible for drug dependence behaviors.[20]

Scientific studies show that not only direct listening, but even the anticipation of the pleasure one feels

____

[20] Hermann Helmholtz. On the Sensations of Tone (Dover Books on Music). Dover Publications, 1954.

when enjoying a melody, also induces the release of dopamine, accompanied by physical reactions in the body.[21]

The feelings, thoughts, and perceptions developed by the psyche determine our adaptation to the ambiance in which we live and to which we relate through processes of a very particular nature, as the result of our life experiences and perceptions of the world. The psyche stores in the unconscious the whole set of information related to the content of our daily experiences, interpretations, and feelings acquired throughout life.

The essence of each of us is continually developed throughout our lives and, in this sense, music enables our moral and spiritual evolution, stimulating a better and healthier disposition in our relations with the world around us.

---

[21] Sir James H. Jeans. Science and Music (Dover Books on Music). Dover Publications, 2012.

7. Music Therapy

Music has a remarkable power to improve our emotional health and to elevate our mood providing a sense of well-being. Thus, music and medicine go in the same direction, seeking to promote the harmony of the human body and general good health.

Since ancient times, traditional Chinese medicine has used music as a valuable therapeutic tool. The benefits range from relieving pain and reducing stress to reducing the use of sedatives and painkillers. However, the use of music in healing processes goes back to the most distant antiquity. Throughout history, from the scarce shreds of evidence that has come to us, it can be identified innumerous reports of therapeutic musical procedures.

Hildegard of Bingen (1098-1179), a German Benedictine abbey, wrote in the 12th century the medical compendium *Physica*, in the period 1150-1158, which was a practical manual of popular healing with herbaceous remedies.[22]   Her holiness was made official in 2012 by

[22]Hildegard Von Bingen's Physica: The Complete English Translation of Her Classic Work on Health and Healing (English) Hardcover – 31

Pope Benedict XVI, who also named her "Doctor of the Church".

At a time when women could not even have formal education, she was a writer, composer, philosopher, legendary healer, poet, and saint. As a musician, she composed 27 symphonic works. In her book, she describes healing methods using plants, elements, trees, stones, fish, birds, animals, reptiles and metals, explaining how to prepare and apply different medicines and their curative use. In his monastery, there was a hospital, where among healing practices she used music therapy too. *Physica*, which means pharmacology, was derived from the practice of monastic medicine over the centuries.

Hildegard's psychotherapy indicates the Five Pillars of health: nurturing the soul, nourishing the body, living healthily (exercises, outdoor living, good habits, friendships, family), enhancing immunity (elixirs, rest, avoiding chemicals, wine, mushrooms), and a regular detoxification (intestinal cleansing, fasting, calendula, sangrias and leeches).

Traditional Chinese medicine is known for its effectiveness in working with natural elements such as the use of herbs and acupuncture, and by uniting the healing

ago 1998 by Hildegard of Bingen (Author), Hildegard (Author), Priscilla Throop (Editor).

power of herbs with the benefits of music. The Chinese character *yào* refers to medicine or drug and is composed of two parts: the upper one indicates herbs, and the lower one is the music radical. However, music, happiness, and herbs form the medical character that exists today in the Chinese language.

Our body is a structure that works rhythmically, governed by the beating of the heart. Our life routine has a cyclic rhythm of activities and sleep. Eastern spiritualist literature tells us about energy channels that run through the human body, called meridians in acupuncture. These constitute 12 pairs, each associated with one organ. A flow of energy must flow freely through the meridians so that the individual keeps good health. Any blockage impairs the harmony for the functioning of the organs, which can evolve into a disease. Where the meridians meet, a great influx of energy occurs, and such agglomerations are known as plexuses or chakras.

In Hindu culture, yogic and occult studies, theosophy and conscientiology, chakras are centers of absorption, exteriorization, and administration of energies in the etheric double of a living organism. These are special energy centers within the body that resemble vortices, closely connected to the nervous system, influencing the nature and quality of the transmission of nerve impulses. They are connected and to the cellular structures through delicate channels of energetic nature. A vast literature can be found today on this subject.[23]

Some specific sounds such as the vowels of the alphabet vibrate in the energetic centers of our body and cause biochemical reactions, which in turn have revitalizing, harmonizing, relaxing and healing effects. Each energy center perceives a specific sound. The main centers encompass the vital (basic) center, the personal center (cardiac), and the impersonal (head) center. Drum sounds stimulate basic chakras and action, while melodious sounds stimulate heart center and affectivity.

According to the Eastern tradition, along the backbone are several of these important centers of energy, associated with our extra-sensory perception, and their improvement gives us a special faculty. Acting as emitters and energetic receptors, the chakras are responsible for capturing the vibrations that benefit us.

An organic imbalance thus reflects some blockage or obstruction that disrupts the free flow of energy through the channels that spread through our body. They are linked to the endocrine glands and thus are determinants of the physical well-being.

---

[23]Chacras e meridians.
http://www.swami-enter.org/pt/text/ecopsicologia/page_36.shtml.

Some beneficial oriental techniques are known for purifying and unclogging the energy plexuses. Among them are the mantras, which represent specific sonorous vibrations specific to each chakra. Such techniques have the effect of refining and purifying them. The tradition highlights the deleterious and toxic effect of alcohol consumption and meat, which are incompatible with the purification of the subtle energetic structures of the energy centers, which can cause serious diseases.

In total, seven are described:.[24]

- *Sahasrara*, similar to a disk (diameter 12 centimeters, height 4 cm), is located in the area of the cerebral hemispheres, under the parietal bone;

-*Ajña*, located in the center of the head;

-*Vishuddha*, situated in the lower part of the neck, up to the level of the clavicles;

- *Anahata*, in the pectoral section of the trunk, between the clavicles and the solar plexus;

- *Manipura*, on the upper abdomen;

- *Svadhisthana*, in the lower abdomen;

---

[24] Os 7 chacras principais dos seres vivos.

- *Muladhara*, in the lower part of the pelvis, between the coccyx and the pubis.

The central meridian is considered a channel of great importance that connects all the chakras in a single set, forming a column. Cleansing the central meridian contributes to enhancing the health of our body.

As far as the degree of development of each chakra is concerned, there are the outstanding faculties for each person, which defines their psychological aptitudes and particularities. For example, a well-developed *vishuddha* indicates faculty for aesthetic perception, as artists in general.

Some sounds are related to the chakras are.[25]

Basic Chakra or Root: The "U" sound activates the forces of initiative, vitality, safety, survival, self-confidence, stability and inner strength.

---

https://www.luzdaserra.com.br/os-7-chacras-principais-dos-seres-viv
os.
[25]A Doutrina Secreta H.P. Blavatsky.   O Livro completo dos Chacras. Ambika Wauters. 1 Jan 2014 by Quarto Publishing (Author), Ambika Wauters (Author);
https://www.eusemfronteiras.com.br/a-relacao-do-som-com-o-corp
o-humano-e-os-chacras-parte-2/ by Silvia Fleury).

Sacral-central or sexual chakra: The "O" sound circularly awakens feelings to integrate the masculine and feminine energy of our being.

Solar Plexus Chakra: The "O" sound stimulates the outer form of our being, starting from an interior perfection. It contributes to the manifestation of fullness and joy in the world.

Heart Chakra: The "A" sound involves the unprejudiced acceptance of all manifestations of affection from which love arises.

Laryngeal chakra: The sound "E" unites the heart and the mind channeling its forces to the external expression.

Frontal Chakra: The "I" sound generates an upward-directed movement that gives the strength of inspiration, leading to new insights and perceptions.

Coronary Chakra: The "I" sound represents undivided unity and pure and unlimited consciousness. (The last two chakras vibrate alike and are the most spiritual ones.[26].

---

[26]C.W.Leadbeater. Os Chakras: Os Centros Magnéticos Vitais do Ser Humano.

In the 1960s a team of Korean researchers conducted a series of studies on the anatomical nature of the meridian system in animals. Mapping was performed, which revealed a system of channels that interconnect the meridians between them, and which also flow into the blood vascular system. The meridian system thus constitutes an interface between the physical body and the etheric body described by Indian medicine.

Music has been used since ancient times to induce a good mood in people. And especially nowadays, with the evolution of the communication tools, this is increasingly part of our daily life, whether in parties, exhibitions, championships, Olympics, celebrations and the most varied collective events.

In the film industry, the musical appeal has a strong influence on the most significant moments in the story to be told. Considering the deep connection that people are increasingly developing with music today, it is even surprising to ignore its benefits in health treatments.

Everyone knows very well the strong emotional effect that it causes to remember past events of our lives with a musical background. In the daily routine, everyone recognizes that after a troubled and dense day of occurrences, some moments of relaxation listening to music that pleases us have a very beneficial and positive effect in building our well-being and mood state. It, therefore, recommended using music as an important part of body health recovery therapy in a variety of situations.

Results from several studies reveal that the impact of music on the nervous system alters heartbeats, breathing, blood pressure, digestion, hormonal balance, temperaments, attitudes, and releases adrenaline. Reactions may vary on each individual but the result is always unique. Van de Wall in his book "Music in Hospitals" points out that sound vibrations cause contractions and movements in the arms, hands, legs and feet.[27]

Already at the times of the music of the great war was used in hospitals to help restore the good mood of soldiers with post-traumatic stress disorder.[28] Noting the positive effect of this, an effort began in the search for developing new techniques and procedures with the aid of skilled musicians to achieve non-musical goals and objectives. The ultimate goal was to achieve harmony between body and mind by attuning to appropriate sounds.

Since then this has been practiced, although still timidly, in many cases of recovery of the physical and emotional health of patients with some type of trauma. It is not uncommon to see reports in the news of people visiting

---

[27] Music in hospitals Front Cover Willem Van de Wall, Russell Sage Foundation, 1946 - Music therapy.

[28] E.A. Baratella. Música e Musicoterapia: Uma Linguagem da Alma. Empório do Livro, 2008.

hospitals, costumed and in groups, in playful activities to amuse and cheer adults and children recovering from painful treatments.

Good humor affects and restores people's good mood. However, even though the profession of a music therapist is not new, it is still practically neglected today in conventional health treatment procedures.

In the first half of the 20th century, Willem van de Wall developed important research in music therapy that contributed significantly to musical education and shaped the practice of hospital musicians. Professional harpist, choral director and music education teacher, throughout his life he wrote numerous articles and several books advocating the structured and controlled use of music in institutions including schools, psychiatric hospitals, general hospitals and prisons.[29]

According to the definition, music therapy is the use of music by the therapist in a structured process to facilitate and promote communication, relation, learning, mobilization, expression and physical, emotional, mental, social and cognitive organization to develop potential and develop or retrieve individual functions so that it can

---

[29]Willem van de Wall: Organizer and Innovator in Music Education and Music Therapy Alicia Ann Clair, George N. Heller George N. Heller Journal of Research in Music Education   Volume: 37 issue: 3, page(s): 165-178 Issue published: October 1. 1989.

achieve better intra and interpersonal integration and consequently a better quality of life.

Since music therapy is a therapeutic intervention, based on the use of sound characteristics directed to living beings, in a music therapy procedure it is sought to select the sound-musical stimuli to be used that may be more effective in the treatment of a given individual. It is crucial to use specific vibrational forms of sound energy that can act effectively on the energy system that may be unbalanced in a living organism.[30]

As we all know, music can influence a person's state of mind in a very personal way. When hearing that song that we love we feel momentary well-being. When listening to a beautiful unknown melody that pleases us, we enjoy moments of unusual enlightenment.

The inner effect, at the psychosomatic, organic and cellular level, has had many interpretations, and several reports have appeared on the response to stimuli that can be detected by special receptors installed in people, animals, and plants.

The concept of the Mozart effect was introduced in 1991 by the French researcher Dr. Alfred A. Tomatis, who believed that good polyphonic music could promote

---

[30] R. Benenzon. Teoria Da Musicoterapia. Summmus Editorial 2018.

healing of a variety of diseases and brain development. Since then several reports have appeared on the use of music with beneficial results in plants and animals. Farmers have opted for classical music to improve plant cultivation, to help cows to produce milk and even to produce bananas and grapes.

In a music therapy procedure, the sonorous stimulus assimilated by the patient submitted to the treatment is transformed into sensations and emotions that are very particular, beneficial and positive to achieve organic balance. If one considers that music is a way of expression of the human unconscious, the depth of the relation music-psyches' is something very complex and little known.

In this sense music can be placed as a determinant path of a therapeutic process, in which it can also contribute positively to psychological treatment to facilitate the expression of the subject, allowing emotional associations and the sublimation of the unconscious drives.

Music therapy thus refers to the clinical use and based on positive evidence of musical interventions to achieve individualized goals, within a therapeutic relation, conducted by an accredited professional. It is the use of music to improve people's quality of life.

The music therapist uses music and all its physical, emotional, mental, social, aesthetic and spiritual facets to help clients improve their health. Consequently, health treatments are now shifting from a simple procedure of attacking only the symptoms of integrated medicine. Each day new studies show that both the emotions and the psychological side and the state of mind of each one participate together in the well-being of the person.[31]

Music therapy has also been increasingly sought and developed to achieve non-musical goals. Significant progress has been reported in cases of children with autism.[32] Besides, psychiatrists have used music therapy as part of the treatment with encouraging results, finding evidence that this can make their patients feel better, help to relieve stress and progress. As revealed by scans with advanced nuclear magnetic resonance imaging (MRI), music can affect both sides of the brain simultaneously.

The complexity of the music, which combines melody, words, rhythm, timbre, with all the richness of sounds and frequencies of a musical phrase, concerning the effects that it can introduce as complementary therapeutics for recovering our physical and mental health represents a fertile field of studies, still quite unknown. Results of

---

[31]. M. Chagas. Musicoterapia. Mauad Editora, 2015.
[32] Betsey King. Music Therapy: Another Path to Learning and Communication for Children in the Autism Spectrum. Future Horizons, Apr. 2004.

investigations with advanced techniques pointed out to the existence of a musical lobe in the brain, as well as the activation and stimuli in various regions of the brain produced by music. This implies effects on memory, emotions, muscle control, vision, hearing, and speech, among others. It has been observed that some Alzheimer's patients with speech and word articulation problems can sing musical excerpts.[33]

However, with the continuous evolution of knowledge about the functioning of the brain, music therapy has been gaining increasing importance in neuroscience. The more we learn about how music works, the more it will be possible to enhance its effectiveness on the recovery and maintenance of our body's health. A central issue in music therapy, however, is to identify what is most important and useful to benefit a patient under treatment. It takes a lot of knowledge to decide what is best in each case, and in which of them is recommended musical intervention.

It is interesting to observe the rhythmic operation mechanism of our body and all living beings, which follow an uninterrupted sequence of processes that goes on indefinitely. Just look at ourselves and see the rhythm of our breathing and heartbeat. Music is an art that explores

---

[33] E. Ruud and E.R. Vera Bloch Wrobel. Caminhos da musicoterapia. Summus Editora, 1990.

the rhythmic sound manifestation, enriched with the harmony of the composition, and that uses infinitude of combination and mixture of different frequencies tempered with the timbre and mode of execution of each component, being this vocal or instrumental.

In speaking, we momentarily express our disposition in a way affected by our intimate mood, and thus, our way of pronouncing words sounds more like a ditty charged with emotion. Also, each person, with its language and peculiar way of verbal expression, has a litany with peculiar intonation, typical of his speaking and discoursing, and this implies a musical aspect that changes even within the same country, where the musical preferences reflect the regional characteristics.

Several benefits with proven efficacy have been observed in therapeutic musical procedures, improving health without harmful effects, provided that carried out in a controlled way. Besides, to enhance our mood state and disposition, it has also a very positive effect on our concentration and ability to develop coordinated reasoning. This is highly recommended in cases of marked stress, depression, anxiety treatments, migraines, and treatment of chronic pain in general.

In recent decades there has been a growing interest in the use of music as an intervention for hospitalized patients. Several studies demonstrate the ability of music to reduce anxiety and positively attenuate the physiological reactions caused by stress. According to a comprehensive survey, conducted to test the hypothesis that surgical patients who listen to music during preoperative waiting have lower stress levels, the results are encouraging and stimulate therapeutic usage.

A critical and categorized evaluation was made to assess the effectiveness of music during normal care in invasive and unpleasant procedures, taking as measurement parameters anxiety, satisfaction, pain, mood and vital signs. [34] The data indicate that music heard with headphones significantly reduced anxiety, and improved mood, tolerance, social interactions, attention, and physical disposition in the patients.

Music therapy applied in children has also produced good results, in addition to developing a better learning capacity. In dealing with emotions, it can explore the most various forms of expression, whether using only experimental music or melodies with lyrics, which makes it possible to convey a poetic meaning with strong emotional content. Dance can also be introduced together with music therapy, which allows, among other benefits, to improve motor coordination and body expression.

---

[34]Cooke M., Chaboyer W. Achluter P. & Hiratos M. The effect of music on preoperative anxiety in day surgery. (2005) Journal of Advanced Nursing 52(1), 47–55.

A research on the comparison of rhythms between language and music has shown that the prosody of the spoken language of culture can influence the structure of its instrumental music.[35] This provides an empirical basis for the claim that speech vocabulary accentuation leaves a mark on the music profile of a culture.

The reason is seen as simple: if music is based on words, and words have different rhythmic properties in different languages, then it would not be surprising if the musical rhythm reflects the linguistic rhythm. Thus, when composers elaborate their works, the linguistic rhythms to which they are accustomed, consciously or unconsciously, strongly influence their artistic creations.

A cultural brand also imposes itself, in which the younger composers are influenced by the music of their compatriots, and this, in turn, is influenced by the music that these composers listened as children, as folk and folk songs, whose rhythms bear the regional mark of their language texts.

Nowadays medicine has been practiced with a holistic approach, involving patients and families with the

---

[35] Aniruddh D. Patel, Joseph R. Daniele. An empirical comparison of rhythm in language and music. The Neurosciences Institute, 10640 John Jay Hopkins Drive, San Diego, CA 92121. USA Received 3 September 2002; accepted 1 October 2002, Cognition 87 (2003) B35–B45.

methods of health care. Alternative therapies have become an adjunct to traditional medicine. Among these, music therapy is a low-cost alternative that is easy to administer and is very beneficial to patients. There are several recommendations suggested, such as allowing patients to select the type of music to be played. No musical selection works best for all people in all situations. In the following are some reports of successful experiences of musical intervention as a complementary therapy.

Hospitalization causes a lot of anxiety in some patients, which increases, even more, when patients wait for a surgical procedure. Music therapy was recommended, for example, to reduce the psychophysiological effects by inducing relaxation, attenuating anxiety, helping to control heart rate and blood pressure in patients awaiting cardiac catheterization.[36] Interesting enough is the fact that, in general, women experience a higher level of anxiety in these cases than men.

A study on the use of relaxing music to dampen the noise level in nursing home dining rooms has shown a significant calming effect, which reduced agitated behaviors particularly among residents with severe

---

[36]Hamel WJ. Intensive Crit Care Nurs. 2001 Oct;17(5):279-85 The effects of music intervention on anxiety in the patient waiting for cardiac catheterization.

cognitive impairment.[37] The presence of noises such as loud music, shouting, people talking loudly or dragging furniture, generated symptoms such as excitement, irritability, distrust, and dissatisfaction in practically all patients. With music, it has been observed a progressively reduced stress threshold among most patients.

In neurology, aphasia is the weakening or loss of the power of capturing, manipulating and sometimes expressing words as symbols of thoughts, due to injuries in some brain centers. A study was conducted on a new form of language therapy to treat aphasia, called Melodic Intonation Therapy, which involves the intonation of sentences in such a way that the pattern intoned is similar to the natural prosodic pattern of the sentence when it is spoken.[38] The results indicated that the use of music is very beneficial in stimulating less developed language areas of the brain as well as recovering some damage in the cerebral hemispheres.

After an evaluation of the effects of music therapy in patients with mechanical ventilation (breathing through

---

[37] Jan Cioddaer and Ivo L. Abraham.   Effects of Relaxing Music on Agitation During Meals Among Nursing Home Residents With Severe Cognitive Impairment   Archives of Psychiatric Nursing, Vol. VIII, No. 3 (June), 1994: pp. 150-158.

[38] Robert Sparks, Nancy Helm, and Martin Albert. Aphasia Rehabilitation Resulting from Melodic Intonation Therapy. Cortex Volume 10, Issue 4, December 1974, Pages 303-316.

devices), it was recognized that music therapy is a more effective nursing intervention in reducing patients' anxiety than a rest period.[39] However, the greater or lesser effectiveness of music to act as an anxiety-reducing agent is dependent on the type of music used, the patient's preferences, and his/her interest in music.

A study was designed to verify whether music or its combination with therapeutic suggestions in the operative period could improve the recovery of patients undergoing hysterectomy under general anesthesia.[40] The data were analyzed through a visual analog scale of symptoms such as nausea, vomiting, intestinal function, fatigue, well-being and duration of hospitalization, considered as indicative of progress. It was observed that on the day of surgery, patients exposed to music in combination with therapeutic suggestions required less analgesic rescue. i.e., more effective analgesia on the first day after surgery, and could then be mobilized sooner after the operation.

---

[39]Heart Lung. 2001 Sep-Oct;30(5):376-87. Effects of music therapy on anxiety in ventilator-dependent patients. Wong HL1. Lopez-Nahas V, Molassiotis A.; Linda Chlan, Effectiveness of a music therapy intervention on relaxation and anxiety for patients receiving ventilatory assistance. Heart Lunge 1998;27:169-76.

[40] U. Nilsson, N. Rawal, L. E. Unestahl, C. Zetterberg and M. Unosson. Improved recovery after music and therapeutic suggestions during general anesthesia: a double-blind randomized controlled trial. Acta Anaesthesiol Scand 2001; 45: 812–817.

A survey of preterm infants in neonatal intensive care units has shown that, in delivering, music is statistically significant and clinically brings important benefits. [41] Lullabies for preterm infants transmit the human voice and provide a language stimulus with important long-term consequences for future learning, as well as to reduce stress and stimulate the critical period of growth, to promote bonding with parents and to facilitate neurological communication and development.

The limbic system is a region made up of neurons, and is the unit responsible for processing and controlling emotions in the human brain and social behaviors. It contains various structures, the hypothalamus, the hippocampus, and the amygdala, which act together to create simple, complex emotions that, through the nervous system, work to help people express and convey thoughts, ideas, and feelings.

The hypothalamus is a small structure, but it plays a key role. This alerts when it is time to sleep, eat and drink, sending signs like fatigue, hunger, and thirst. Neuroscience research shows that emotions evoked by music can modulate limbic and paralimbic activity and brain structures. These affect the neuroaffective mechanisms,

---

[41] Jayne M. Standley. A Meta-Analysis of the Efficacy of Music Therapy for Premature Infants. Journal of Pediatric Nursing, Vol 17, No 2 (April), 2002.

whose dysfunctions are related to emotional disorders. Therefore, a better understanding of the correlation between the emotions stimulated by music and the neural processes can lead to more effective use of this in therapies.[42]

A study was done to investigate the effect of three non-pharmacological nursing interventions, i.e., relaxation, music, and the combination of relaxation and music on pain after gynecological surgery in a total of 311 patients aged 18 to 70 in five hospitals of the Midwest of the United States. [43] The data collected provided evidence that strongly supports music therapy and relaxation in the pharmacological treatment of pain after surgery, thus improving the effectiveness of health services. It was observed that both the sensation of pain and the postoperative distress were significantly reduced, which contributed to reduce the side effects of the medication and to accelerate the recovery of patients.

In obstetrics, the control of labor pain and the prevention of suffering are major concerns of both clinicians and their clients. Research has been developed to

---

[42] Koelsch S1. Trends Cogn Sci. 2010 Mar;14(3):131-7. DOI: 10.1016/j.tics.2010.01.002. Epub 2010 Feb 10. Towards a neural basis of music-evoked emotions.
[43] Good M1. Anderson GC, Stanton-Hicks M, Grass JA, Makii M.. Relaxation and music reduce pain after gynecologic surgery. Pain Manag Nurs. 2002 Jun;3(2):61-70.

evaluate the efficacy of non-pharmacological methods used to alleviate pain and reduce labor pain. Several methods were studied, such as music, acupuncture, massage, hypnosis, aromatherapy, and audio analgesia, which presented evidence of generalized satisfaction among the majority of patients.

Audio-analgesia is the use of auditory stimulation, such as music, noise, or ambient sounds to decrease the perception of pain. Its use is popular for pain relief during dental work, or after surgery, or even in other painful situations, such as in childbirth.[44] Music provided a more attractive distraction because, with the help of a music therapist, where the patient can control the volume and make her own choice, for example for ambient sounds, to enter into a relaxed or hypnotic state, which facilitates the labor of delivering.

The conclusion is that, as there are no known disadvantages in the use of music or ambient sounds during childbirth, as well as because no adverse effects of audio analgesia are known, this seems to be an acceptable option in which usage can be encouraged.

Bronchoscopy is an endoscopic procedure used to visualize the tracheobronchial tree, with a diagnostic and

---

[44]Simkin P1. Bolding A. Update on nonpharmacologic approaches to relieve labor pain and prevent suffering. J Midwifery Women's Health. 2004 Nov-Dec;49(6):489-504.

therapeutic purpose, which can be done through rigid or flexible equipment.[45] Tests have been performed on adult patients in a US hospital to determine whether nature's sound therapy can reduce pain and anxiety. Some panels with nature scenes were placed at the bedside, and patients were given a tape of nature sounds to listen to, before, during and after the procedure. Patients from another group were offered neither the nature scene nor the sounds.

The results showed that the chances of better pain control were higher in the patients who received the musical procedure than in those who did not have the same treatment and received only the narcotic medication. Older patients and patients in better health reported significantly less pain when they have listened to music. The study concludes that distraction therapy significantly reduces pain in patients undergoing painful invasive procedures.

Hematologic neoplasms are malignant tumors originating from blood cells, bone marrow, and lymphatic system. High-dose therapy with stem cell transplantation is a treatment commonly used to treat such cases and is a procedure that causes certain psychological distress.[46]

---

[45]Diette GB1. Lechtzin N, Haponik E, Devrotes A, Rubin HR. Distraction therapy with nature sights and sounds reduces pain during flexible bronchoscopy: a complementary approach to routine analgesia. Chest. 2003 Mar;123(3):941-8.
[46]Cassileth BR1. Vickers AJ, Magill LA. Music therapy for mood disturbance during hospitalization for autologous stem cell

Tests performed in some patients with hematologic malignancies who were treated with music therapy by trained therapists showed that there was a significant reduction in the combination of anxiety and depression in several acute medical contexts.

The musical rhythm is an important factor in the temporal structure of music and has a profound effect on the human motor system and behavior. Several kinds of research that have been recently developed provide evidence that the interaction between rhythm and physical response can be effectively harnessed for specific therapeutic purposes in the rehabilitation of people with movement disorders.[47]

Dyslexia is the learning disturbance and difficulty in understanding the reading and recognition of the correspondence between graphic symbols and phonemes, as well as in the transformation of signs written into verbal signs. There is a great deal of evidence suggesting that the language and reading problems experienced by dyslexics are caused by deficiencies in various sensory, cognitive and motor processes.

transplantation: a randomized controlled trial. Cancer. 2003 Dec 15;98(12):2723-9.

[47] Thaut MH1. Kenyon GP, Schauer ML, McIntosh GC. The connection between rhythmicity and brain function. IEEE Eng Med Biol Mag. 1999 Mar-Apr;18(2):101-8.

Some theories point to the idea that fundamental problems derive from abnormal neurological time or temporal processing, and thus it is suggested that the temporal processing capacity can be improved through training. [48] It is concluded that music training, which requires very precise timing skills, may offer a valuable means for the development and improvement of the temporal processing capacity for dyslexic children.

A controlled trial was conducted at a hospital in Belgium to evaluate the effect of a musical exercise program on the mood state and cognitive function in patients with dementia.[49] The patients underwent physical training for three months consisting of daily physical exercises supported by music. The results were compared with another group of control patients who received an equal amount of attention through daily conversations. The results indicated a beneficial effect of the music-based exercise program.

A study was conducted comparing music and non-music conditions in the treatment of children and

---

[48] Katie Overy. Dyslexia, Temporal Processing, and Music: The Potential of Music as an Early Learning Aid for Dyslexic Children. Psychology of Music Volume: 28 issue: 2, page(s): 218-229 October 1. 2000.

[49] Ann Van de Winckel, Hilde Feys, Willy De Weerdt. Cognitive and behavioral effects of music-based exercises in patients with

adolescents with autism, considering variables such as the number of subjects in treatment sessions, participation, selection and presentation of music, researcher's discipline and patient's age. The conclusion is that all musical interventions, regardless of purpose or implementation, have a beneficial effect on treatment.[50]

In outpatient surgery, surgical procedures are performed with general, local, regional or sedation anesthesia, which require short-term, non-intensive postoperative care. This waives hospitalization for allowing discharge in a few hours after the procedure. However, it is known that this can also create significant anxiety in patients. A prospective study has assessed whether music can influence anxiety and the need for a perioperative sedative in outpatients.[51]

Perioperative is the term used in Medicine for the period that goes between, since the surgeon decides to indicate the operation and communicates to the patient until

---

dementia. Volume: 18 issue: 3, page(s): 253-260 Issue published: May 1. 2004.

[50] Jennifer Whipple. Music in Intervention for Children and Adolescents with Autism: A Meta-Analysis. Journal of Music Therapy, Volume 41. Issue 2, Summer 2004, Pages 90–106, https://doi.org/10.1093/jmt/41.2.90.

[51] Caroline Lepage, MD, Pierre Drolet, MD, Michel Girard, MD, MHPE, Yvan Grenier, MD, and Richard DeGagne, MPs. Music Decreases Sedative Requirements During Spinal Anesthesia. (Anesth Analg 2001;93:912–6).

the latter returns, after discharge from hospital, to normal activities. Measured anxiety levels were assessed and compared with other patients who did not hear music. The conclusion is that patients listening to music require less medication to achieve a reasonable degree of relaxation.

Several studies show that music is widely used to improve well-being, reduce stress and distract patients from unpleasant symptoms. Although there are wide variations in individual preferences, music seems to exert direct physiological effects through the autonomic nervous system.[52]

This effectively reduces anxiety and improves the mood of patients in intensive care units and patients undergoing painful procedures, be they, children or adults. Music therapy is a low-cost intervention that helps reduce surgical, procedural, acute and chronic pain and contributes to improved empathy, compassion, and patient-centered care.

Finally, there are countless cases of successful situations that indicate music therapy as a valuable mechanism to aid in the recovery of good health and improve the mood state of patients. This is not expected to be advised absolutely in all situations, but the positive

---

[52]Kemper KJ1. Music as therapy. South Med J. 2005 Mar;98(3):282-8.

results stimulate further studies and the development of this technique.

The music therapist is a health professional who guides a treatment where music is used within a therapeutic relationship to meet the physical, emotional, cognitive and social needs of people of all ages, whether they are healthy or are facing some illness. This initially seeks to assess the unique needs of its patients. The treatment environments are quite varied, and include clinics, hospitals, nursing homes and even schools.

Music therapy, also called musical medicine, is based on two fundamental methods, i.e., that of listening (receptive method), and that of creation, performed by singing or else by playing musical instruments (active method). Basically, there are two types of the receptive method. One of them refers to relaxation music therapy, indicated for the treatment of anxiety, depression and cognitive disorders. The other is recognized as receptive analytical music therapy, recommended by analytical psychotherapy.

Music therapy is thus a process-oriented practice, instead of being based on the excellence of the patient's musical performance, where individuals are encouraged to actively participate in musical interventions to achieve functional therapeutic results. Interventions can include singing, dancing, or performing movements in a choreography submitted to the rhythm of the music, or then by playing a variety of instruments which are important tools of a music therapist and must be chosen specifically based on the needs and objectives of patients. In addition, one can still do meditation by listening to music.

The first stage of a musical medicine treatment process necessarily involves a functional assessment of the individual's abilities and needs, conducted through sound stimuli and observing the responses obtained in motor, sensory, emotional, behavioral and social skills.

A music therapy session is planned in view of a series of important factors for the effective achievement of a successful treatment, which includes several important factors, such as the patient's physical health, his ease and ability to communicate, his cognitive skills, the emotional well-being, and obviously a clear definition of what are the goals to be achieved.

After a careful and comprehensive analysis of the different points of attention, the music therapist thus decides whether to use the creative or receptive method. In the first case, he acts to produce music actively, which can involve simply free musical improvisation or the composition of a harmonious melody, which can be done through singing or playing musical instruments, including a rhythmic performance of beats and strokes with a wide variety of percussion instruments, such as drums, bells, metal tuning forks, etc. In the receptive method, the therapist offers listening experiences to induce the relaxation of a single patient or a group. At the end of the session, patients can discuss thoughts, sensations, ideas and feelings evoked by listening to music.

Guided meditation is another modality in which the person meditates following instructions directed by a professional in a session or class held with the use of music, or else by means of some rhythmic stimuli. This can also be done using audiovisual techniques or a mobile device. Meditation can also involve singing or the repetition of mantras and prayers. Among the intended benefits are the reduction of anxiety, stress and depression.

As music therapy seeks to reach all aspects of the mind, body, brain and behavior, it can be indicated as an auxiliary procedure in a variety of treatments, for example, to help in the rehabilitation of patients after a stroke, a traumatic brain injury, or in chronic diseases. such as Parkinson's or Alzheimer's, as well as emotional health problems (sadness, anxiety and depression), as well as physical rehabilitation, pain control and more complex cases of recovery from brain injuries.

The patient does not necessarily need to have any musical ability to benefit from music therapy. In addition, all styles of music can be beneficial. The preferences of each person and the need for treatment help in choosing the most appropriate type of music, a process that usually includes choosing a song that has some deeper meaning for that person, and the way it can affect or awaken positive emotions. Music therapy can also offer help to improve the communication performance of those who have some difficulty in expressing themselves through words.

When working with children, it is observed that there are certain instruments that a music therapist tends to use more often than others, either because of the ease of execution, which encourages the participation of children, or because of the most appropriate shape and size, for example, a set of small bells and drums, which can be richly colored and decorated with letters of the alphabet, as well as small stringed instruments.

It is essential to continuously assess the progress made to reach the desired goal at the end of the treatment. This involves the permanent collection of data, records and relevant documentation of the steps taken, as well as the review of the intended objectives, allowing flexibility for changes and new adaptations, if necessary. In addition, collaboration with other health professionals during the process is essential, which allows to deepen the procedure's effectiveness in a very significant way.

It is important to note that there are several different ways of performing sound therapy, where a variety of different benefits are sought. However, among the various possible modalities, not all are necessarily musical. For example, tuning fork therapy uses specially tuned devices to apply specific vibrations in different parts of the human body, used as an auxiliary method to relieve tension and promote the patient's physical and emotional balance. Similar to acupuncture, the treatment aims at specific stimulation in specific regions of the body using sound frequencies, instead of needles. Studies suggest that this type of therapy can effectively help relieve muscle pain.

Psychoacoustics is the science that refers to the scientific study of people's sound perception, and analyzes the psychological responses associated with different types of sound. An important topic in the psychology of music is the study of the human ear and the way the brain reacts to musical perception. It seeks to understand the physiological mechanisms responsible for transforming the sound stimulus into auditory sensations. Music can involve anything from a simple distraction to the mind or a means to slow down the rhythms of our body and change our mood, which in a way also influences behavior.

A field of studies also of great interest in musical medicine is the neurological effect of the so-called binaural beats or sounds, a procedure that involves a method to stimulate the brain to a specific state using pulsating sound, aiming to stimulate the brain waves to align with the frequency of the beat. The goal is to seek to induce an improved focus of attention in the patient, leading to a state of trance, relaxation and sleep. This method offers promising new perspectives in some treatments, such as controlling and reducing anxiety, relieving pain, and also to improve behavioral problems in children and adolescents. Research in the field of music medicine has shown that adequate sound stimuli can help regulate activity in specific regions of the brain that are involved in controlling emotions.

Another type of music therapy procedure that has been widely discussed involves the display of images with musical accompaniment. These are used as a starting point to stimulate sensations and emotions, which allows directing the discussion with problems that are somewhat related to that situation. The music therapist can then prescribe musical medicine combined with the presentation of images in a programmed context and directed to be enjoyed by the patient even outside the office or treatment environment. Studies have shown that this method, when applied in a way that explores the musical rhythm more strongly, allows to favor the execution of movements, which helps in the treatment of patients with some type of motor-coordination difficulty.

The therapeutic use of music and its effects at the neurological level are not yet fully understood but, because of the results achieved, the prospects are encouraging. In dealing with emotions and feelings, the possibilities of benefit with its use have found increasing recognition among health professionals. With the advancement of knowledge about the functioning of our brain, music therapy has gained more and more important in health treatments. As Hildegard de Bingen said, "health is harmony between body, soul, and spirit".

Music has the power to change our mood suddenly and profoundly, harmonizing our feelings and behavior with our inner disposition, giving us a sense of euphoria and well-being, which positively affects our mind, our soul and our body, and which provides us a decisive way to achieve better health.

8. The Sound as Therapy

Quantum Medicine is a form of alternative medicine that represents the result of the union of medical knowledge with the sophistication of technology. The Indian physician Deepak Chopra, a resident in the United States, coined the term in his book *The Quantum Healing*, which has become a reference in treatments that encompass body and mind.[53]

In his book are presented results of his studies on *Ayurveda*, which in Sanskrit means, the Science of Life. This is a traditional Indian practice that is based on the idea that the cells of our body can be modified by thought. From this, at least in principle, anyone could cure himself of diseases, provided he attains harmony between body and mind.

In quantum medicine, it is suggested that a clinical intervention should be done with the use of devices that act both in the elaboration of diagnosis and in the

---

[53] Quantum Healing: Exploring the Frontiers of Mind-Body Medicine Chopra, D. ISBN 978-0307569950, 2009, Random House Publishing Group
https://books.google.com.br/books?id=0SPiUOU_fIQC.

treatment. Nowadays, an increasing number of followers of this modality is observed, since it is believed that this allows a more general description of the general health of a person, as well as predisposes the body to find the organic balance more effectively.

Since then the word *quantum* has never been so fashionable. It turns out that many people consider that the view of modern physics that matter and energy are equivalent implies directly that all humans are formed by energy and connected through it, and that this implies quantum behavior.

Some even cite Einstein's famous equation, $E = mc^2$, which shows the equivalence between matter and energy as a justification for claiming that everything can be quantum. They even speak of *quantum energy*, which makes no sense at all! The indiscriminate use of the word quantum is not well regarded by the scientific community.

There is a gratuitous mixture of concepts in which it is affirmed that vibrations, resonances, and waves imply quantum manifestations, and from there, the quantum cure. By assuming a conception that absolutely everything in the universe occurs via vibrations, it is assumed that the quantum must be in everything. It rather would be better to use than the term "vibrational."

In physics, a quantum is the minimum quantity of any physical entity present in an interaction. From there, physical property is said quantized when it can assume only discrete values that are integer multiples of a quantum. For example, the energy levels of a particle confined within an atomic system are quantized, which means that it can only assume certain discrete energy values. There are forbidden values. The electronic energy levels in the materials are quantized. On the other hand, in classical physics, any particle can have any energy.

Quantum physics is used predominantly to deal with problems at the atomic level, where size scales are vanishingly small, and so the treatment of interactions between particles requires adequate tools in these tiny dimensions. The amounts of energy involved are very small, as in the spacing between the electronic levels of an atom. Today we still do not have any method of registration that can confirm that the interaction between body and mind is quantum in nature. For now, it is pure speculation, and any statement of that is superficial and dubious.

However, it is imperative to make it very clear that there is no intention here to attack the foundations of Quantum Medicine or criticize its practice. Rather, the goal is to alert to the careless and abusive use that is seen in these days of the word quantum.

The recognition of the vibrational aspect of many natural phenomena has attracted the attention of researchers, who are beginning to sketch a greater interconnection between Physics and Medicine, particularly in therapeutics. The vibrational therapies are intended to deal with the energetic and vibrational part of the human body.[54]

When someone gets sick, with quantum therapy he or she tries to identify disharmonious information in the body to achieve positive changes in health. The law of universal attraction is invoked, where thought plays a fundamental role in self-suggestion and the uptake of positive energies. However, the more positive things we are cultivating in our thoughts and feelings, the more positive things we bring into our lives.

We often hear that words have power, and the more bad things you say, the more negative things will be with you. This is the law of attraction. By focusing on positive ideas, and speaking only positive things, we are more predisposed to find more joy and prosperity in our lives. As we spread love, we will receive more love. It is the law of action and reaction. As Master Chico Xavier said, "it is necessary to sanctify the thoughts and purify the feelings."

---

[54]R. Gerber. Medicina vibracional: uma medicina para o futuro. Cultrix, 2002.

The scientific method is a logical and rational order of steps by which scientists come to conclusions about the world around us. This represents an organized way of discovering something, seeking to organize the thoughts and procedures, so that the answers found to the questions originally proposed have credibility and can be accepted as proven scientific truths. Any scientist, anywhere in the world, as long as he has the proper conditions, should be able to confirm the results of a study done by others by following the correct steps of a research procedure.

Scientists use observations, hypotheses, and deductions to build up their conclusions. Observation is the first step in deciding the nature of the research. The hypothesis is the answer to a question raised at the beginning of the investigation, thus anticipating a description of what is expected to be achieved at the end of the process. Prediction is the specific belief about the scientific idea: If the hypothesis is true, then the prediction will be confirmed. The experiment is the set of procedures used in all steps of the research to try to raise the data needed to answer the initial question. The analysis is a detailed survey and study of what happened during the experiment. Finally, the conclusion is the answer found to verify that the hypothesis was correct. The steps of the scientific method are:

- observation/research,

- hypothesis,

- experiment,

- analysis,

- conclusion.

It is also possible to discriminate:

- independent variable: it is a part of the experiment that will be tested;

- dependent variable: is what is observed in response to the chosen independent variable;

- control: it is the part of the experiment where the independent variable is not included and allows comparing the different results of the experiment.

The procedures adopted following the scientific method minimize the influence of the researcher when testing a hypothesis or theory. If the results of the experiments confirm the hypothesis initially pointed out, it can be considered as consonant with natural law. If, on the other hand, they do not confirm the hypothesis, it must be rejected or modified.

It may even happen that a discovery or new experience comes into conflict with a long-held theory. Therefore, even if a theory seems perfect and incorruptible so that it is finally accepted as scientific truth and accepted by all, it needs confirmation, which usually comes from experimental results, and hence it can be considered as a valid description of the observed events.

Thus, a new theory needs and must be tested, before entering into the role of scientific truths. It may happen, however, that a long-held accepted theory may suddenly show itself at odds with new observed results, and so it is threatened to be dismissed as an incorrect description of reality, but still provides fairly reasonable results within a range of measurable parameters.

This is what happened, for example, with classical mechanics, completely valid and acceptable in events observed in our daily activities at low-speed regime, but whose predictions fail in the regime of high speeds or the world of the sub-atomic particles. In this way, classical physics is valid only at distances much greater than the atomic scales, whereas the predictions of quantum mechanics are valid in all scales of dimensions.

Some theories have been discarded in the face of new experimental evidence. In cosmology, for example, the ancient geocentric model, in which Earth was considered at the center of the universe, remained for many centuries as irrefutable, but it was eventually replaced by the heliocentric model of the Copernican system, in which the sun is placed in the center of the planetary orbits. This theory was finally accepted when measurements of the movements of the planets ended up confirming the new model.

The scientific method, therefore, seeks to minimize the influence of the scientist on the outcome of an experiment by preventing a biased posture from influencing the acceptance or rejection of a hypothesis. Many times the scholar may have preference or repulsion for a particular hypothesis, which he would very much like to be accepted or refused. Thus, the latter may decide to ignore or exclude data that do not support the hypothesis or even seek evidence in systematic errors that lead to a direction that has a decisive influence on the hypothesis raised initially, resulting in a certain form of data control.

It is therefore of great importance that all data be treated in the same way. Indeed, inappropriate treatment of the data can also compromise the validity of the results in the analysis of a hypothesis.

A hypothesis represents somehow a limited view in a cause and effect relation to very specific situations and also reflects our state of knowledge about a particular subject, even before an experimental work of verification has been performed. A consolidated scientific theory represents a set of hypotheses that have already been verified several times and in different situations, preferentially including experimental tests.

A scientific theory, once confirmed as true, then becomes part of our view and understanding of the universe and a starting point for further inquiry, and this will remain unchanged until discovery or a new phenomenon comes to challenge what was consolidated

Nowadays, much is said about Quantum Vibrational Therapy, as a fundamental part of future medicine. This is considered as an alternative form of treatment for physical and emotional disorders, which seeks to deal with causes and effects together. Quantum therapy is considered an energy therapy and then acts in a holistic process that aligns body, mind, and spirit.

The recommendation is that quantum therapies should be used as a complement to orthodox medicine to boost its results. It is imperative that the individual reaches his mental, physical and spiritual balance so that healing becomes possible.

From modern physics, a certain amount of matter has an equivalent in energy. From this, some draw a direct conclusion that all human beings are formed by energy and thus interact with each other by energetic vibrations. But from there to quantum therapy, the leap is huge.

However, for many, quantum vibrational therapy is controversial because of its distorted interpretations of modern physics, and is even recognized by the scientific community for lack of coherence in the scientific terms it adopts. Although there is a background of truth in the mention of the vibrational aspect of the matter, this does not necessarily imply quantum behavior for everything.

The controversy revolves around the fact that macroscopic objects such as the human body or individual cells are too large to have inherently quantum properties, such as interference, diffraction, quantum entanglement, and the collapse of the quantum mechanical wave function describing the motion of a particle.

Some have pointed out that there has often been a misuse of the word quantum. A misleading concept that the vibrations of the universe are quantum and that they connect all beings in this context is abused and unscrupulously explored. It is a somewhat pretentious statement that tends to place all phenomena of enormous complexity in a commonplace.

This is a careless way of arguing for laymen, for those who do not understand the subject. Some interactions have nothing of quantum. There is no quantum energy! There is quantized energy or quantum of energy.

Currently, bioenergy represents a field of studies in which a method of treatment based on the energetic aspects of living organisms is sought. Biological organisms are believed to emit and absorb energy at various frequencies. It is interesting to note that in the millennial Eastern cultures there are records of the belief that our bodies have energy channels that operate at various frequencies to heal and maintain health.

Several well-known oriental healing modalities are based on the energetic functions of these energy channels. Nowadays new healing methods have been developed in the field of alternative medicine, seeking a link between the ancient methods used in Eastern traditions under a new point of view pointed by the science of the West.

German biophysicist Fritz Albert Popp of the University of Kaiserlautern claimed in the 1970s that all cells of living organisms can store and emit particles of electromagnetic radiation, called bio-photons. He believed he had discovered the cure for cancer. In his studies, Popp hoped to be able to predict which chemicals are carcinogenic. Investigating the effect of radiation on living organisms he was fascinated about a phenomenon called photo-repairing: by illuminating a living cell with wavelength 380 nm UV light, to destroy its DNA, he believed it was possible to repair a disease in one the only day! The hypothesis raised at that time was that a carcinogen acts to block photo repairing. However, this never was duly substantiated.

Still, in the 1970s, Popp built a photomultiplier machine that detected light waves emitted by cucumbers and potatoes. At first, he believed that this had something to do with photosynthesis, but the radiation detected was coherent, i.e., formed by waves of the same frequency and direction of propagation which maintained a constant phase relationship between each other.

In his interpretation, Popp spoke of equivalence with a set of tuning forks that reverberated together. He pointed out that the molecules in the cells responded to certain frequencies and that the photon frequencies of the light waves caused a variety of vibrational frequencies in the molecules of the body.

Throughout the 20th century, several theories and reports of experimental observations appeared on the existence of energetic fields around living organisms, citing morphic fields, mitogenic radiation, and electric fields, defining forms, growth, structures, and regeneration. There were also reports of experiments with plants grown from seeds that revealed the presence of electric fields resembling the adult plant. In the book *The Secret Life of Plants,* by Peter Tompkins and Christopher Bird, in the 70s, are presented several reports of studies conducted in different places around the globe, studying the relations between humans, plants and the surroundings.[55]

The sensibility of living beings thus began to be discussed at that time on the level of telepathy and parapsychology, with surprising but questionable interpretations. Impressive genetic alterations have also been reported in small living organisms when passing electric currents and applying high voltages.[56]

Particularly in the last decades, several reports have appeared from several researchers, in many places around the world, discussing results of observations that wave vibrations are responsible for the synchrony of cell division and for sending chromosomal instructions to the whole body.

The physicist Herbert Frohlich (1905-1991) at the University of Liverpool, who won the Max Planck Medal, acknowledged that some kind of collective vibration is responsible for getting the proteins to cooperate with one another and to follow DNA instructions, and predicted that certain frequencies (now called "Frohlich frequencies") can be generated by vibrations in proteins. A vibratory signal

---

[55]Peter Tompkins. The Secret Life of Plants. Harper Row, Publishers, Mar 1989.
[56]Don Campbell. The Mozart Effect: Tapping the Power of Music to Heal the Body, Strengthen the Mind, and Unlock the Creative Spirit. Avon Books, 1997.

would be how the smallest activities of the proteins, such as the work of the amino acids, would be executed, as well as the mechanism to synchronize the activities between the proteins and the whole system.

The Italian researcher Renato Nobili, from the University of Padova, presented a study on the functioning of the brain and the informational nature of human thought, where he discusses the mechanisms that cause the oscillatory activity of specialized populations of neurons.

He argues that this activity, which underlies the general mammalian memory strategy, may explain the extraordinary ability of the human brain to process large amounts of information very quickly. The author further believes that this kind of parallel processing of information can be implemented in integrated optoelectronic devices.

A vibration that travels through a given medium with the passage of a mechanical wave, transfers energy incisively to all the atoms in the region, which in turn communicate to their neighbors the disturbance received. Each structure, with its shape and dimensions, allows the excitation of characteristic vibrational modes.

In a string instrument, for example, there is a harmonic series that corresponds to the so-called vibrational modes or standing wave patterns that can be produced by vibrating each string at specific frequencies.

These are defined by the length and the tension to which it is subjected, as well as its mass and density.

When a string vibrates at one of its resonant frequencies, a maximum of energy is transmitted to the body of the musical instrument, which in turn transmits it to the surrounding air. The instrument box acts in this way as an acoustic amplifier, which conveys the perceived vibrations to the air.

The sound thus peculiarly flows into the ambiance, corresponding to the timbre produced by the instrument, defined by its shape and construction. A bass string placed on a violin will not have the same effect since this latter is not suitable for vibrating at the resonant frequencies of the bass string.

The size of a structure influences which vibrations it can withstand more easily. For example, a severe earthquake struck Mexico City in 1985, and while many medium-sized buildings were razed to the ground, lower structures and large skyscrapers remained virtually intact.

It turns out that the higher a building is, the more sensitive it is to low frequency seismic vibrations, which is equivalent to longer wavelength waves. In April 1883 a brigade of soldiers marched along the Broughton Suspension Bridge in England, which caused the structure to rupture and the bridge collapsed when the bridge was vibrated in one of its natural frequencies upon the rhythmic strokes of the march of the platoon.

All physical structures have a so-called natural frequency of vibration, characteristic of their construction, density, composition and the way mass and rigidity are distributed. When a pulsating external force acts on a given structure in such a way that its oscillation frequency equals exactly the natural frequency of the object, the so-called resonance phenomenon takes place.

By vibrating in its natural frequency under the action of an external stimulus, the tendency is a considerable increase in the amplitude, which can lead to the rupture and disintegration of the whole system. In machines such as pumps, turbines, and electric motors, for example, the resonance can amplify the small vibrations occurring during the machine operation and therein cause severe damage.

By intoning a musical note with a specific frequency, an opera singer can break a wine glass. The sound level need not be too high, just having the right frequency is enough, which needs to match exactly the natural frequency of resonance of the glass. When this happens, the vibrations have increased oscillations, which cause the glass to shatter. Each body, each object, has its resonant frequencies.

The frequency range of mechanical vibrations in material media may be beyond the reach of human hearing. This is the case of infrasound and ultrasound, which are below or above the human audible range (20-2000 0 Hz), respectively. Acoustic resonance is a phenomenon that occurs when systems amplify intercepted sound waves whose frequencies correspond exactly to their natural vibrational frequencies.

In general, objects have more than one resonance frequency and possess what is called harmonic vibrational modes. A structure vibrates more easily in the natural frequencies of the harmonic series. This represents a fundamental aspect of the design and construction of a musical instrument. The body of the instrument is the resonant cavity that responds strongly to the frequencies it perceives belonging to its harmonic series, whether are these produced by vibrating strings, tubes or membranes.

A resonator is a device or system designed to exhibit resonance, i.e., to vibrate easily at well-defined frequencies, i.e., the harmonic modes. The oscillations in a resonator can be electromagnetic or mechanical. Acoustic musical instruments use resonators designed to amplify specific sound waves.

Cavity resonators, where sound waves are produced by air vibrations, are known as Helmholtz resonators. The geometric shapes, therefore, are not the only determinants of the vibrational properties of a resonator. Another important contribution arises from the chemical constitution, temperature, the nature of the fluids filling the cavity and their viscosities, i.e., whether these are liquids or gases. The geometric shape of the resonant cavity indeed has a great influence on the vibrational modes. For example, the length determines the frequencies of the harmonic series, while the width influences the rate of dissipation of the energy of the vibrations.

The resonance frequency thus depends both on the dimensions of the cavity as well as on the properties of the medium it contains. In acoustic cavities filled with fluids, gases or liquids, the change in the elastic characteristics of the medium found in the path of the sound waves causes a reduction in the amplitude of the resonant frequencies.

In musical instruments, the cavity resonators have the function of modifying the sound to improve specific frequencies, as in the body of string instruments, and the tubes of wind instruments. On the other hand, some can act as noise mufflers, such as in the exhaustion system of cars and motorcycles. Others may also have the function of removing combustion products from turbines and engines.

The guitar resonator is a device for guiding the harmonics of the guitar strings by an electromagnetic field.

This resonance effect is caused by a feedback loop and it is applied to drive the fundamental tones and some musical ranges to infinite sustain.

Natural phenomena such as earthquakes, large bursts of explosions and thunder, or even the wind, are capable of causing severe structural damage by resonance. Not all accidents of this type imply that resonance has occurred, but when it is the case, the effects can be catastrophic.

Each structure has a natural frequency. For example, our eyes have a resonance frequency of about 50 Hz, slightly above the beginning of the human audible range. Our rib cage has a resonance frequency in the range 50-100 Hz, which coincides with low-pitched sounds.

In a seismic shock, the waves intercepted by the structures put the whole set into vibration. Thus, when the frequency of these waves is close to the resonant frequency of the structure, the effect can be catastrophic, and even lead to the rupture and collapse of the shape. For example, skyscrapers with height above 100 m have an extension equivalent to a wavelength $\lambda = 100$ m, which for a wave traveling at about 340 m/s equals a frequency $f = v/\lambda = 3.4$ Hz (vibrations per second).

Thus, when the seismic waves have this very frequency of vibration, there occurs the resonance, which entails an increase of the amplitude of vibrations that can cause the collapse. Smaller structures, such as buildings below 20 m, have an associated parameter $\lambda = 20$ m, which, for $v = 340$ m/s, gives $f = v/\lambda = 17$ Hz. That is, the higher structures have a higher risk of damage to seismic waves of lower frequencies, while the lower constructions otherwise suffer greater damage to seismic waves of higher frequencies.

However, both transverse and longitudinal waves are there in seismic waves. These depend upon both the modulus of elasticity and density of the medium. For seismic waves through the bulk material, the longitudinal or compressional waves are called P waves (for "primary" waves) whereas the transverse waves are called S waves ("secondary" waves). The latter is more dangerous than the former because they have greater amplitude and produce vertical and horizontal motion of the ground surface. The slowest waves, surface waves, arrive last, and they travel only along the surface of the Earth. Certainly, the physical constitution of the soil is also very important in determining the effect of the vibrations that occur during an earthquake, for example, the existence of rocky or sandy soils.

To minimize the effect of resonance, the natural frequency of the object in question should be changed to less expected value among those that may occur more easily. Possible measures include adding more rigidity to the structure, increasing its natural frequency, adding more mass, reducing the natural frequency or increasing damping to change the natural frequency of vibration of the structure to a frequency where the forces are much weaker and, as a consequence, have a lesser effect.

In general, all structural systems have multiple natural frequencies of vibration. If it is forced in any way to vibrate at any of these frequencies, the response will be amplified, resulting in higher tension and vibration levels than expected, thus implying a dangerous situation. Excitations might occur over a wide range of frequencies encompassing one or more of the system's natural vibration frequencies. Or, this may occur in another specific tonal excitation including some higher-order vibrational harmonic modes where some of the resonant frequencies can be close to a natural structural frequency.

All buildings have a natural period of oscillation, which is the time required to complete a vibration, i.e., to naturally swing back and forth. The soil also has a specific natural frequency. A bed of hard rock has natural frequencies greater than softer sediments. If the period of movement of the ground coincides with that of a building, it will suffer the largest oscillations, and as a consequence, will suffer the greatest damage. Thus, a resonance frequency of any system is the frequency at which the maximum amplitude oscillation will occur.

Sonar is an equipment used to make underwater or atmospheric sweeping using acoustic vibrations, which can be very low (infrasonic) or very high (ultrasonic). The operation can be passive, picking up sounds, or active, emitting pulses and collecting echoes. Sonar works like radar but uses sonic pulses instead of radio waves. The device emits a sound pulse that, when encountering an obstacle, returns to the transmitter, which allows mapping the region.

Dolphins also use a complex tracking mechanism using ultrasound. These emit an explorer click, lasting less than a thousandth of a second, which is progressively adjusted until an eco-response is obtained that provides information for identifying the object in question. Their operating frequency is between 20-120.000 Hertz. A treatment called Lithotripsy is used to break down kidney stones using shock waves, which avoids aggressive surgical intervention. With this technique, one can use sound waves to generate clashes in a sequence that act as beats to break apart the kidney stones.

On the other hand, in vibrational medicine one seeks to use, detect and analyze vibrations in the human body, specifically to restore health.[57] Music, for example, has long been used for the treatment of diseases, such as

---

[57] Ivette Catarina Jabour Kairalla e Maristela Pires da Costa Smith. A musicoterapia na medicina quântica. Revista InCantare, 0(0), 2014.

neuropathy and depression. This seems to have been known to the ancient Greeks and Romans. Nowadays, with the fast advancement of the technology, which allows generating a wide range of acoustic frequencies with high precision and control, besides recording high-quality images, there is increasing interest in the use of vibrational therapies as a therapeutic adjunct.

On the other hand, plants are also complex multicellular organisms, quite sensitive to external stimuli through the epidermal cells. Plant growth is considered to be the sum of cell proliferation and subsequent stretching. This is vital for the evolution of the plant as a whole as well as for the creation of new organs that give quality to the organism in development.

Sound is an external factor that has a great impact on plants and can promote or even suppress growth. In addition to external stimuli, such as moisture, nutrients, temperature, light, heat, and wind, there is evidence from experimental results that sound waves with specific frequencies and intensities affect plant growth, such as seed germination, root lengthening, plant height, callus growth, enzymatic and hormonal activities, and gene expression. However, this effect may also be negative. It is the field of studies of cellular biology.

Since the 1950s several studies have appeared reporting on the effect of music and sonic devices on plants. The results indicated that sounds emitted with frequencies between 125-250 Hz had the effect of making some genes related to plant growth more active, and conversely, a negative effect was observed with lower vibrations, around 50 Hz. Experiments carried out to investigate the effect of sound and different musical styles on plants showed the best growth results when using classical music.

Other stimuli such as sound fields, supersonic sound, electromagnetic fields, microgravity, and mechanical vibrations also showed a varied impact on plants.[58] Living organisms can sense and respond to physical stimuli. Some vegetables exhibited positive effects for melodic trails. While sounds of only a few kHz and sound levels below 100 dB are beneficial on the chrysanthemum culture, high frequency and high-intensity sound otherwise have a detrimental influence. In humans, 100 dB represents the pain threshold for the sound level.

Although the mechanisms by which sound waves stimulation influences the development of plants remain unclear, it is known that some specific frequencies and

---

[58]Md Emran Khan Chowdhury, Hyoun Lim, and Hanhong Bae. Update on the effects of sound waves on plants. Research in Plant Disease, 20:1–7, 03 2014. Tanto a frequência quanto a intensidade parecem influenciar o desenvolvimento de algumas plantas Dorothy Retallack. The Sound of Music and Plants. DeVorss and Co., 1973.

intensities have significant effects on various biological, biochemical and physiological activities of vegetables.

Results of recent studies conducted in the USA at the University of Buffalo and the Hauptman-Woodward Medical Research Institute have been published in the journal Nature Communications 10, 1026 (2019). They report evidence that proteins in living things vibrate continuously, like a violin's strings or the tubes of an organ. According to the authors, "it is fascinating to think that a true symphony of vibrations exists in living organisms." Such motions allow the proteins to change rapidly and to form new bonds to perform critical biological processes and functions such as oxygen uptake, cell repair, and DNA duplication.

Vibrations in living beings have both mechanical and psychological effects, which depend on the duration of exposure, posture, points of contact and applied forces. These can be either general or local. For instance, vibrations with frequencies up to 500 Hz cause fatigue and worsening of reactions to external stimuli on the human body, when there is prolonged exposure, such as in the operation of heavy machinery and vehicles. These are "vibrations of the whole body."

The spine is the most sensitive part of vibrations when exposed to oscillations in the vertical direction, along the axis of the spine, which can cause severe low back pain.

Pneumatic hand tools, operating in the frequency range 20-40 Hz, can cause damage to the hands, while vibrations at frequencies above 100 Hz are known to affect mostly the fingers.

Ultrasonography is a non-invasive method that uses ultrasound generated by high-frequency waves to map the internal structures of the body via ultrasound imaging. By capturing images in real-time, this technique is very important to analyze the functioning of the organs in a living organism, without causing any harm to the patient. It usually employs ultrasound in the frequency range between 2 MHz and 50 MHz, which are emitted utilizing a piezoelectric crystal transducer, which emits and receives the echoes of the sound waves, transforming them into signals that will be interpreted to generate images. A 3.5 MHz transducer is indicated for deeper examinations, whereas a 7.5 MHz transducer is suitable for more superficial examinations.

Although this is a safe technique, because it does not use ionizing radiation as in radiography and tomography, sound waves can however cause an increase of temperature in the tissues, forming small bubbles of gas in the body fluids, which when collapsed, can release free radicals that cause chemical damage to biological molecules, such as DNA.

Low-intensity acoustic waves are now used in the treatment of erectile dysfunction of vascular origin. These waves accelerate regeneration processes, improve metabolism and increase the blood circulation of damaged tissue. Effective treatment of pediatric patients with burn scars has been done using 3 MHz ultrasound.[59] Since ultrasound also produces thermal effects, the intensity of the radiation applied is an essential factor for the success of any therapy as well as the duration of the exposure.

Besides, are also observed effects such as increased membrane permeability and nerve conduction, vasodilation, analgesia, increased protein synthesis rate and fibroblast activities, increased metabolic rate, the release of histamine and chemotactic agents, increased transport of calcium ions through cell membranes, increased synthesis and elasticity of collagen, among others.

Sound therapy can be practiced in many ways, such as music, singing, dancing, meditation and playing an instrument. In vibrational sound therapy, sounds are used for producing vibrations directed to the brain. Such therapies have a variety of effects on our body such as in blood pressure, relaxation, breathing, pain relief, and anxiety.

---

[59]Eficácia do ultra som de 3 MHz em pacientes pediátricos com cicatrizes, sequelas de queimaduras de segundo a terceiro grau. Área de Cirurgia Plástica Reabilitadora do Hospital Infantil, Córdoba, Argentina: 2006-2012 Blanco MGR, Bencivenga MJ, Jensen LG.

The conventional music therapy is used to meet the physical, emotional, cognitive and social needs of an individual or a group, which employs a variety of activities such as listening to melodies, playing an instrument, writing songs, sometimes accompanied by dance and rhythmic exercises.

It is possible to imagine a near future where sound waves are used in a wide range of therapeutic procedures. Imagine that, in a fictitious and futuristic vision, new sonic therapeutic techniques using musical chords will emerge, based on a harmonization of specific frequencies, with the simultaneous application of a special set of frequencies for composing a particular melodic trail using harmonic triads, for example, for health treatment.

And, like in science fiction movies, a person goes into a cocoon for a therapeutic vibrational treatment, and after some time finally accomplishes the cure of a disease. But of course, for now, this is still pure fiction! And it is worth remembering that until now only the acoustic modes have been mentioned. Besides these, there are also the optical modes, relative to the electromagnetic waves, that carry light and heat.

However, one question that arises is: would it be possible to restore the organic balance in damaged living tissues using vibrations on a level never before imagined? Or, would there be adequate vibrational therapy for recovering an organ with a certain disease, or even for removing aggressive tumors? How to determine which are the most appropriate sonic stimulus, and at what intensity?

Despite some successful procedures in vibrational therapy, there is still a long way to go. The future will tell us. Is this something like quantized vibrational therapy? Quantizing means putting in numerical quantity by adding a numerical value, to put in a scale of discrete values, i.e., quantifying. The concept then indicates a supposed treatment produced with sound waves controlled in intensity and at certain discrete frequencies, limited in number and within a specific range, to promote health or stimulate the development of living organisms, such as plants and animals.

The choice of discrete frequencies involves constructing a regime of vibrational modes that can be identified as important to stimulate the proper functioning of the organs for a given structure, animal or plant. These could be based on the harmonic tonal modes of a musical scale, which defines a specific relation between the different degrees of the scale. One use could exploit, for example, the natural frequencies, to identify characteristic wavelengths compatible with the dimensions in question.

The human body has a maximum length of about two meters, which implies an equivalent wavelength corresponding to a frequency of 170 Hz for sound waves traveling at the speed of sound in the air (343 m/s at 20°C). However, the propagation velocity of the sound depends on the medium. In water, this is about 1,500 m/s and still depends on its purity and temperature. In the fat, this is about 1,430 m/s, in muscles and tissues 1,580 m/s, and bones this ranges from 3,500 to 4,300 m/s. The relation $\lambda f = v$ allows determining the frequency corresponding to each velocity, for a given wavelength λ. Ultrasound is in the range of 30 kHz to 100 MHz, and above it is the hyper sound. So the exact definition of the vibrational regime to be employed depends on each case and it takes a lot of discernment to make the right choice. And this depends on a lot of studies

The sound produced by the vibration of thick strings, such as those of the acoustic bass or cello, gives us a kind of low-frequency itching. If these vibrations can be controlled by amplifiers and other equipment, the combined effect of a set of notes sounded simultaneous, smoothly, is quite peculiar, which can lead us to a state of relaxation and meditation.

Sound therapy performed with the application of higher frequencies, such as higher musical notes, are useful in treatments for tinnitus in the ear, as confirmed by experiments.[60] It has been observed that by applying additional sounds that the ears can perceive, the tinnitus tends to become less noticeable.

A few years ago a project was developed to evaluate the effect of sound on the growth rate of veggies. It has been observed that two different plant species, bean and a flower (impatiens), were affected by sounds of varied frequencies.[61] Due to their rapid growth, environmental conditions were carefully controlled, and the plants were then subjected to different sounds with approximately the same sound intensity.

Pure tones and random noise were used for comparison. Changes in plant growth were monitored every day for twenty-eight days. After the completion of the tests, it was observed that the ideal growth of the plant occurred when it was exposed to pure tones in which the wavelength coincided with the average of the main dimensions of the leaves.

It has been suggested that this is due to the action of friction on airborne particles on the leaf surface caused

[60] H. M. Moir, J. C. Jackson, and J. F. C. Windmill. Extremely high-frequency sensitivity in a simple ear. Biology Letters, 9(4):20130241–20130241. May 2013.
[61] Margaret E. Collins and John E.K. Foreman. The Effect of Sound on the Growth of Plants. 3 Vol. 29 No. 2 (2001) Canadian Acoustics/Acoustique Canadienne.

by sound waves, which removed the layer of stagnant air adjacent, thus increasing the transpiration of the plant.

For beans, growth with random noise was lesser than that observed with any pure musical tonality. The results indicate that the plant growth rate is even higher when they are exposed to pure tones with a wavelength coincident with leaf width, and a higher sound pressure level (above 90 dB).

There was still evidence that there is a correlation between the sound wavelength and leaf size with a resulting increase in sweating. A significant effect was observed between the frequencies of the sound at which the wavelength is equal to twice the size of the leaf.

An article published in New Scientist magazine in 2007 also gives scientific support to the theory that certain types of sound, such as music indeed can improve plant growth.[62] It is suggested that exposure to certain sound wave patterns results in the activation of sound-sensitive genes and the enhancement of their growth. The research, however, indicates that, in principle, any sound can stimulate plant growth.

In one study, plants that were exposed to sounds for six hours a day had more growth than others placed in a

---

[62] New Scientist 1st September 2007 Issue No: 2619.

silent control group. However, a curious fact is that, while music helped plant growing, it seems to be no more effective than non-musical sounds. The exact cause of the effect of music on plants is thus still unclear. It is believed that they may have a sort of mechanical mechanism that responds to pressure.

In sum, in spite of the numerous experiments reported and the innumerable theories that arose discussing the question of the vibratory nature of the functioning of living organisms, much has been speculated dubiously and questionably, relying on concepts created by pure speculation and without scientific proof.

However, the common point of convergence is that vibratory phenomena indeed are responsible for causing effects. Our planet, with its infinity of sounds and noises, imposes influences upon the entire community of living organisms where vibrations are inherent in its dynamic, through the onset of tremors in all possible shapes, structures and forms. For us, the direct effect of these vibrations at a deeper level is unimaginable, many of them being imperceptible to human ears. However, with the use of appropriate equipment, it is already possible to identify major effects related to mechanical vibrations on certain structures. Nowadays new technologies have been increasingly investigated and developed to reduce noise, undesirable vibrations in machines and equipment, as well as to protect buildings against quakes and earthquakes.

The possibilities are therefore almost infinite, and there is much to investigate. Today, with the increasing evolution of computing engineering and the development of new technologies for data collection and transmission, a new and fascinating field of study offers an interesting way to go, with results still unpredictable, where neuroscience allied with technology has a fundamental role.

The therapy of sound interposes itself as an auxiliary mechanism for conquering a healthier life, by allowing us to harmonize our inner universe with the aid brought by the richness of the musical tonalities.

9. The Celestial Music

The therapeutic value of music seems to have been experienced since the earliest antiquity, as identified from the healing rituals of ancient tribes, where priests and healers sang chants to ward off evil spirits and rescue the sick.

Everyone knows the beneficial effects of good music and the well-being enjoyed by listening to pleasing songs that deliver a state of contentment and satisfaction. Who has not ever felt overjoyed hearing an appealing song? Or did experience an exaggerated sentimentality by enjoying a melodic, emotive and expressive soundtrack?

According to spirituality, we are provisionally embodied spirits and prisoners of a physical body with a profound limitation of sensory perception, but which still makes us highly susceptible to the effects of vibrational influences, both positive and negative, that we assimilate through the centers of energetic activity in our body.

Good music contributes to the elevation of spirit, and the more developed the sensitivity, the more enchantment one can enjoy. We are however also easily disturbed and prone to imbalance, when under a strong negative influence. In Alan Kardec's *Book of Spirits*, it is mentioned the importance of music to the soul, as well as the existence of a heavenly sublime melody, present in all divine creation, and unequaled with the earthly.

In the spiritualist literature, there are still countless reports about the celestial music, emitted from the most varied sources, which also include the diverse celestial bodies that compose the Universe. In the book *Our Home*, by André Luiz, it is reported that, in the *bigger world*, beautiful melodies circulate through the public ambiance which stimulates productive service and collective well-being. Some say that if we could hear cosmic music in its fullness, we could perceive the symphony of creation originated from everywhere, coming from flowers, trees, rivers and waterfalls, *the song of the sky and the stars*.

Spiritualists say that celestial music is the divine melody, emanated by the divine creation, which spreads everywhere. Despite the almost absolute vacuum in interstellar space, it propagates in a way that we do not know, which implies orchestrated melodies via mechanisms that we cannot even imagine.

We are evolving beings, far from understanding all the wonders of creation, and our still rudimentary science needs a long way of studies to enable us to reach a minimum level of discernment to recognize and understand an even deeper complexity of vibrational phenomena and all forms of energy in which matter presents itself.

The creative force of the universal intelligence manifests itself in everything with perfect and absolute harmony, and every new discovery of something that gives us a glimpse of the greatness and complexity of the universe provides an overwhelming impression. But today it is still not obvious to a scientist, who seeks to apply the scientific method to everything he studies, to talk about spirituality and naturally accept concepts whose truthfulness rests on faith and the belief that we are contacted by spirits who live in other dimensions.

For many, science and religion or spirituality still do not mix. Yet the beauty of creation can be admired everywhere, whether in the most diversified form of life on our planet or in the little that we can decipher from the universe that comes to us through electromagnetic radiation.

If we are made of flesh and spirit, how does music affect us spiritually? If our lives are deeply influenced by the spiritual world, the way music can affect our spirit connects us in some way with the surroundings through the law of attunement, which can be good or bad. Negative influences also suggest us nasty thoughts and evil tendencies thus driving our vibratory pattern to a lower and animalistic level we still carry in our being, inherent to our condition.

The connotation of enchantment that good music conveys allows us to be more predisposed to good influences and suggestibility to more positive things, whose results surely bring us greater benefit, both organically as well as into our mind, feelings and thoughts. This also gives rise to a more positive and beneficial disposition from our part towards those which are close to us. People, animals, and plants would perceive a more tender treatment on our part, thus enjoying a better mood. That which gives us something good, makes us better, and this is reflected in our behavior and the way we interact with what is around us.

The good vibrations that we experience end up by spreading to whatever is in the immediate vicinity, which in turn will somehow trigger mechanisms of multiplication of good vibes in such unpredictable ways and independently of our will and control. Goodness propagates.

In the wilderness, far from the intrinsic disturbance and perturbation of the great urban centers, we can perceive the sound of nature, from animals, birds, wind, where we identify pleasant intonations that translate all the dynamics of the planet in which we live, with its immense variety of creatures and sounds.

A large diversity of sounds reaches us from everywhere, uninterruptedly and incessantly. Whoever sings, when cultivating good feelings, transmits to the surroundings a milder emotional climate, which pleases and encourages good predispositions in the listeners, which contributes to the elevation of feelings and sensations in everyone.

By using a musical instrument, the expression of emotions can be further enriched with new tonalities, where harmony can reach higher levels, translating the effort and intention of the performers to contribute to the spiritual elevation of the ambiance.

If we believe in an almighty God, our search for connection with the divine should not be restricted to temples or moments of prayer alone. These, no doubt, generally allow a better focus for our thoughts and feelings, but if we seek to cultivate the discipline of mind and body as well as of sensations and thoughts, in most of our daily routine, we become more apt to receive the good vibrations that the universe continually provides, as well as distributing a higher elevated vibratory pattern, as an antenna radiates the vibrations with which it is fed.

In Buddhism, mindfulness is one of the seven factors of enlightenment. This goes beyond simply paying attention to things, and many people have adopted it as a mode of meditation. It is pure consciousness, free from judgments and concepts and self-reference. Some psychologists have adopted meditation techniques as a therapeutic practice. This can help us to realize the illusory nature of things and to break ties of self-attachment. Genuine mindfulness requires discipline, which can begin with breathing and progress to everything, but if our daily practice is singing, this can work too. An experience of enlightenment is the awakening spiritually, which exposes our thoughts and feelings.

Music manifests itself as a mechanism that enables us to achieve sublimation by providing moments of overjoy and good emotions, pleasant sensations, well-being, and ecstasy. In the collective aspect, musical manifestations unite people around a strong emotion shared by a group, such as in sports competitions, musical shows, parades, carnivals, celebrations, dance exhibitions, etc.

Even in the ancient times, rhythmic music was used to coordinate rowing movements on boats, or, when in the sorrowful times of slavery, to impose a work rhythm on the labor. It was a way of disciplining a group with a language that could be understood by anyone, even without words.

In the past, the search for the correspondence between the planets and harmonic modes has been the subject of investigation of many different scholars in different places and at different times. In ancient Greece,

Pythagoras spoke in Music of the Spheres (*Musica Universalis*) to refer to the connection of the divine harmony between the macrocosm and microcosm.[63] This incorporates the Pythagorean concept that mathematical relations express harmonies that manifest themselves in numbers and sounds with a pattern of proportion. In his theory of the Harmony of the Spheres, Pythagoras proposes that the Sun, the Moon and the planets emit their *humming* based on their orbital revolution, imperceptible to the human hearing, but in frequencies defined by harmonic modes similar to musical ones.

It would not be audible music, in the ordinary sense of the term, but rather a Pythagorean harmonics and philosophical concept which considered the proportions in the movements of the celestial bodies as a form of music.

In the Pythagorean school, the numbers assumed fundamental importance, and everything was supposed to be designed numerically. They tried to relate the elements of the universe in proportions of numerical harmony. It was believed that the celestial spheres were related to the proportions of integers similarly to harmonic musical intervals, as symbols of the divine perfection of the cosmic order.

---

[63] Jamie James. The Music of the Spheres: Music, Science, and the Natural Order of the Universe. Copernicus, Apr 1995.

At that time were known the planets Mercury, Venus, Mars, Jupiter, and Saturn. In designing a seven-note musical scale, the Pythagoreans attempted an equivalent proportion for the relative velocities between the planets. Thus, they associated Saturn with the note B, Jupiter with C, Mars with D, Sun with E, Mercury with F, Venus with G and the Moon with A. This did not imply an audible interval audible to human ears, but rather an abstract concept of the structure of the cosmos. Since then numerous stories have appeared discussing the concept of celestial harmonic theory, which lasted until the Renaissance.

Numerous reports have emerged over time indicating definite proportions in planetary orbits based on the numerology of the Pythagoreanism. In the 16th century the German astronomer and mathematician Johannes Kepler, author of the laws of planetary movements, also seems to have assimilated the concept of the Music of the Spheres in developing his studies of astronomy.

In Kepler's view, the celestial spheres were geometric spatial regions containing the planetary orbits as spinning spheres, similar to the Aristotelian view. In his book *Harmonices Mundi* he sought to explain the astronomical proportions in terms of harmony.

In establishing his celestial-harmonic relations, however, he abandoned the Pythagorean attunement as the basis for musical consonance and adopted musical reasons based on geometry, which allowed him to relate the musical consonance with angular velocities of the planets.

Kepler used the term harmony not referring strictly to the musical definition, but in a broader context that encompasses the congruence in nature and the functioning of both celestial and terrestrial bodies. For him, musical harmony was derived from angles. In his book, he wrote about regular polygons, the congruence of figures, the origin of harmonic proportions in music, and the harmonic configurations in astrology and the harmony of the movements of the planets.

The concept of harmony and aesthetics in antiquity sought to reflect the celestial harmony for the preservation of good social order and equilibrium. The concept of beauty was based on the harmony of forms and harmony of proportions, which spread out widely among all arts, including fashion and architecture.

Although no writing of Pythagoras has come to us, the first definite formulation of a scientific theory of the Pythagorean system of musical intervals appeared in the 4th century BC in Plato's *Timaeus*.

The view at that time was that the universe presented characteristics of the harmony and perfection of the mathematical proportions for the establishment of the cosmic and universal order. There was a belief that the divine mind descends through hierarchies into the human body. The microcosm would then have been created in correspondence of the macrocosm.

The Music of the Spheres remained for a long time as a paradigm of perfect harmony and reflection of the perfect balance of the cosmic order and divine creation. In Rome, Cicero also spoke of the Music of the Spheres and the musical cosmos. The concepts of harmony and cosmic regularity based on mathematical proportions went through the middle ages until the 15th century, with profound influence on the great thinkers and all eminent scientists and theologians of that time.

On the other hand, for some, the cosmic music is the origin of the celestial hierarchies. It is the triumphal melody played by cherubim's and seraphim's in the celebration of the "rites of mystical marriage of the ninth mystery" that Beethoven recorded in the magnificent chorus of the 9th symphony. It has already been said that mankind cannot experience the high spiritual exaltation of this until it has learned to build universal fraternity.

For Beethoven, the musical poem was the expression of spiritual freedom, of the emancipation of the soul, and freedom of the spirit from all physical and material limitations. It meant freedom to wander freely through the higher spiritual planes, to contact celestial beings who inhabit these planes and to hear the glorious celestial music.

According to the spiritualists, "...the musical vibration can stimulate the spirit, provoking sensations of a higher level that puts us in tune with the superior, awakening the Divine essence that sleeps in each one of us."

By recognizing ourselves as evolving, limited, and imperfect beings, we can try to see the world a little beyond logic and reason, and appreciate a more intuitive aspect of learning and knowledge. We cannot rationally explain everything, and when we become aware of our ignorance and limitations, we open our minds to assimilate new influences from the unknown. The musical effect on the human being, according to Plato, is directed to the brain, to the blood and the soul.

In the 12th century, Hildegard of Bingen wrote in her book, *Scivias*, "... words are the body and music the spirit. And so words symbolize the body, and joyful music indicates spirit, heavenly harmony shows the divinity, and the words, the humanity of the Son of God."

Good music thus exerts the beneficial influence of the good and the beautiful and can touch the hearer deeply, for it strikes the heart directly, develops the sensibility, and enables us to elevate the noble nature of our moral impressions.